For more information . . .

This booklet is only one of many free booklets for people with cancer. Here are some others you and your loved ones may find useful:

- *Chemotherapy and You*

- *Eating Hints for Cancer Patients*

- *Taking Part in Cancer Treatment Research Studies*

- *Pain Control*

- *Radiation Therapy and You*

- *Taking Time: Support for People With Cancer*

- *Thinking About Complementary and Alternative Medicine: A Guide for People With Cancer*

- *When Your Parent Has Cancer: A Guide for Teens*

- *When Someone You Love Is Being Treated for Cancer: Support for Caregivers*

- *When Someone You Love Has Advanced Cancer: Support for Caregivers*

These booklets are available from the National Cancer Institute (NCI). To learn more about the specific type of cancer you have or to request any of these booklets, visit NCI's website (http://www.cancer.gov). You can also call NCI's Cancer Information Service at 1-800-4-CANCER (1-800-422-6237) to speak with an information specialist.

Coping With Advanced Cancer

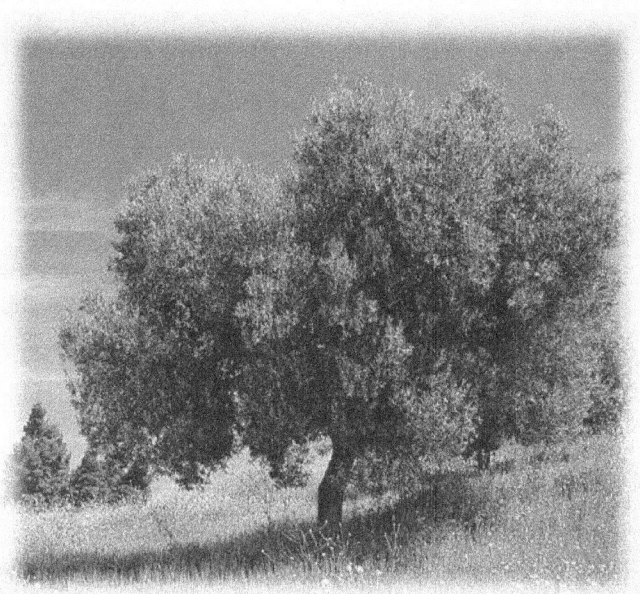

"What lies behind us
and what lies before us
are tiny matters
compared to what lies
within us."

—*Ralph Waldo Emerson*

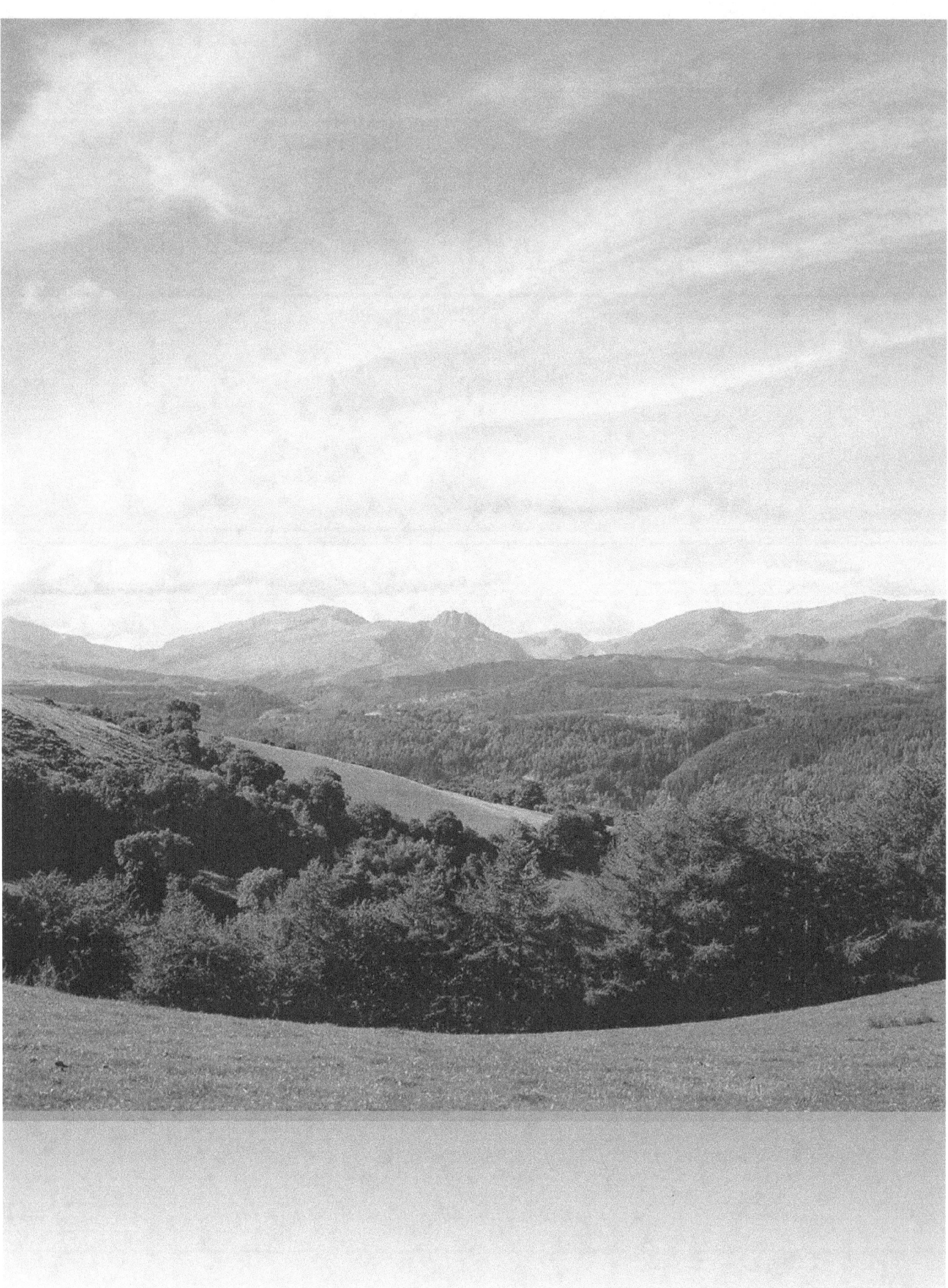

Contents

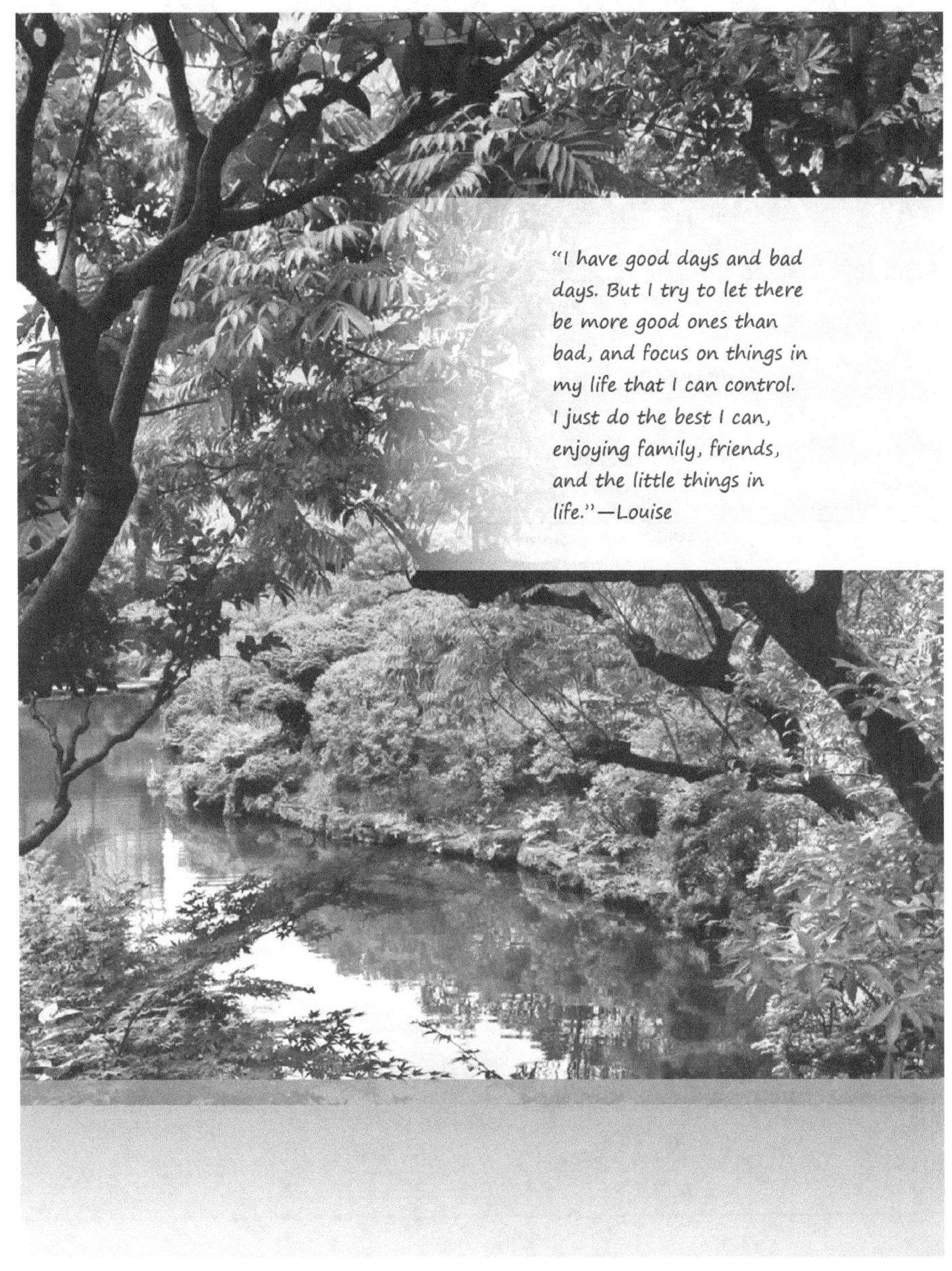

"I have good days and bad days. But I try to let there be more good ones than bad, and focus on things in my life that I can control. I just do the best I can, enjoying family, friends, and the little things in life."—Louise

CHAPTER 1

About This Booklet

You've struggled with the **diagnosis**, treatment, and maybe the **recurrence** of cancer. Now doctors may have told you that you have **advanced cancer.** They may have said that your cancer is not responding to treatment and that long-term **remission** is no longer likely. Or they may have said they have run out of **standard treatment** options. However you learn the news, it can be devastating to you and your loved ones. Often it's hard to believe or accept at first.

Having advanced cancer can bring anxiety and uncertainty to your life. But some people with advanced cancer live far longer than expected. And remember, you are still in control of your choices and actions. Having an advanced disease can be a time of personal growth. It can even be a time of second chances. Many people say they started to see life in a new way after learning that their cancer had progressed despite treatment. They realized the importance of making the most of each day.

This booklet stresses four main points:

- Learning more about ways you can help yourself may ease some of your concerns.

- Your treatment may change, but as always, you deserve to ask for and receive good medical attention from your health care team and support from your caregivers.

- It's important to talk about your worries, frustrations, and problems, and get support from others. In fact, it may be one of the best things you can do for yourself.

- As your medical care changes, you still have many choices. You can choose the way you wish to live each day.

> "There are lots of things I still want to do, but I know that I may not be able to do them the way I planned. But that doesn't stop me from trying to achieve them in a different way." —Millie

Reading This Booklet

No two people are alike. Some chapters of this booklet may apply to you, while others may not. Or some may be more useful later on. As you read this booklet, choose the parts that are right for you. Share it with your family members and loved ones. They may find it helpful to read it with you. Keep in mind that this booklet is for you, an adult with advanced cancer, and the people close to you. For other information for a parent or loved one of a child or young person with cancer, see the NCI booklet, *Young People With Cancer.* Your friends and family members may also want to see the NCI booklet, *When Someone You Love Has Advanced Cancer.*

Above all else, try to remember that you are still in charge of your life. It may be hard to do this with all that you are going through. You may have trouble coping with your feelings from time to time. Or you may be grieving that your life has gone a different way than you had hoped. It's natural to feel negative at times. You'll have ups and downs. We hope this booklet will help you. Our goal is to help you stay in control as much as you can, and make the rest of your life fulfilling and satisfying. You can still have hope and joy in your life, even as you cope with what lies ahead.

CHAPTER 2

Making Choices About Care

People have different goals for care when dealing with advanced cancer. And your goals for care may be changing. Perhaps you had been hoping for a remission. Yet now you need to think more about controlling the spread or growth of the cancer. Your decisions about treatment will be very personal. You will want to seek the help of your loved ones and health care providers. But only you can decide what to do. Your desire to avoid future regrets should be measured against the positives and negatives of treatment.

Questions you may want to ask:

- What's the best we can hope for by trying another treatment? What is the goal?

- Is this treatment plan meant to help side effects, slow the spread of cancer, or both?

- Is there a chance that a new treatment will be found while we try the old one?

- What's the most likely result of trying this treatment?

- What are the possible side effects and other downsides of the treatment? How likely are they?

- Are the possible rewards bigger than the possible drawbacks?

It is important to ask your health care team what to expect in the future. It's also important to be clear with them about how much information you want to receive from them.

Comfort Care

You have a right to comfort care both during and after treatment. This kind of care is often called **palliative care**. It includes treating or preventing cancer symptoms and the side effects caused by treatment. Comfort care can also mean getting help with emotional and spiritual problems during and after cancer treatment. Sometimes patients don't want to tell the doctor about their symptoms. They only want to focus on the cancer. Yet you can improve your quality of life with comfort care.

People once thought of palliative care as a way to comfort those dying of cancer. Doctors now offer this care to all cancer patients, beginning when the cancer is diagnosed. You should receive palliative care through treatment, survival, and advanced disease. Your **oncologist** may be able to help you. But a palliative care specialist may be the best person to treat some problems. Ask your doctor or nurse if there is a specialist you can go to.

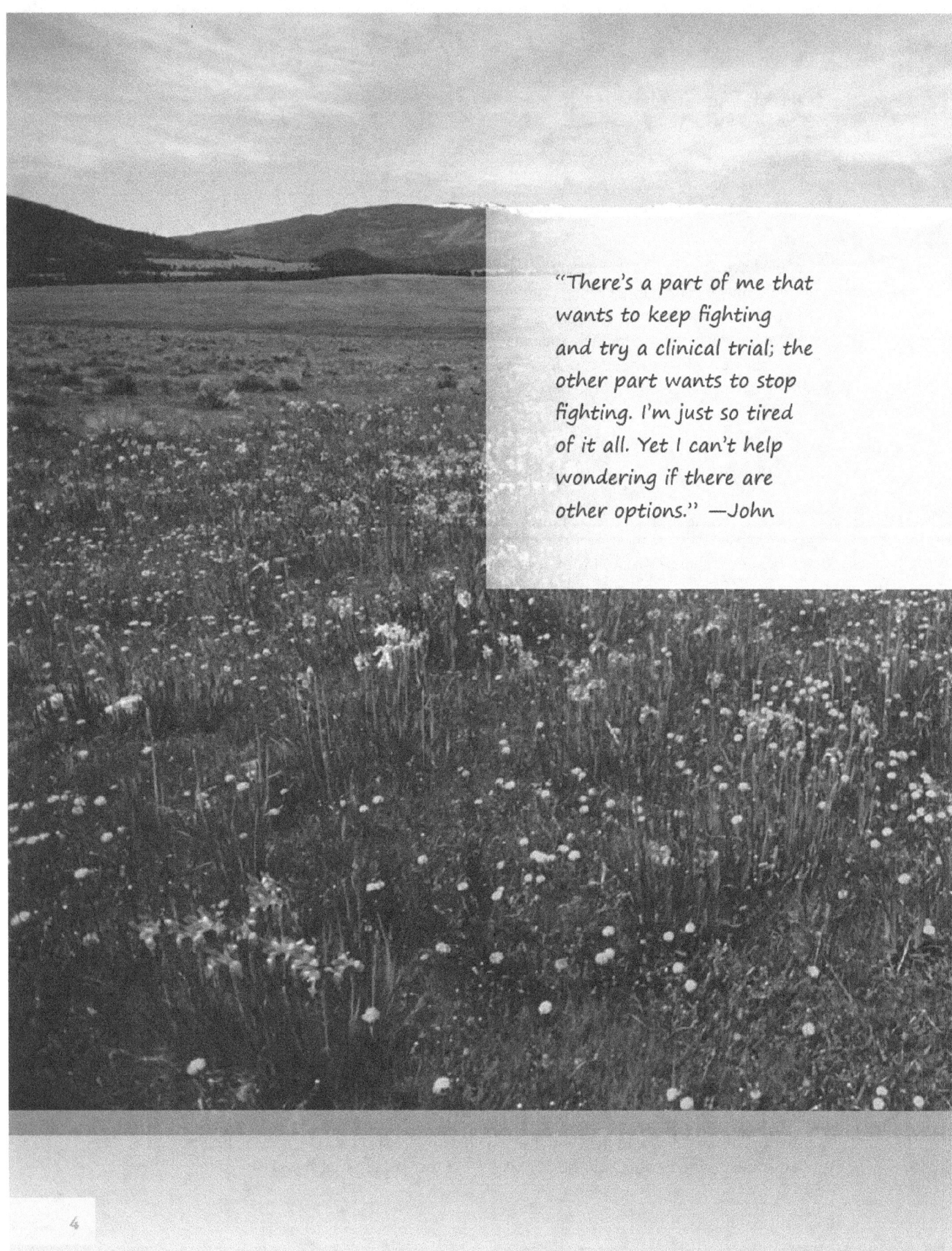

"There's a part of me that wants to keep fighting and try a clinical trial; the other part wants to stop fighting. I'm just so tired of it all. Yet I can't help wondering if there are other options." —John

Your Choices

You have a number of options for your care. These depend on the type of cancer you have and the goals you have for your care. Your health care team should tell you about any procedures and treatments available, as well as the benefits and risks of those treatments.

Options include:

- Clinical trials
- Palliative radiation, chemotherapy, or surgery
- Hospice care
- Home care

Many patients choose more than one option. Ask all the questions you need to.

Try to base your decision on your own feelings about life and death, and the pros and cons of cancer treatment. If you choose not to receive any more active cancer treatment, it does not necessarily mean a quick decline and death. It also does not mean you will stop being given palliative care. Your health care team can offer information and advice on options. You also may want to talk about these options with family members and others who are close to you.

Clinical Trials

Treatment clinical trials are research studies that try to find better ways to treat cancer. Every day, cancer researchers learn more about treatment options from clinical trials. The different types of clinical trials are:

- Phase 1 trials test how to give a drug, how often it should be given, and what dose is safe. Usually, only a small number of patients take part.
- Phase 2 trials discover how cancer responds to a new drug treatment. More patients take part.
- Phase 3 trials compare an accepted cancer treatment (standard treatment) with a new treatment that researchers hope is better. More treatment centers and patients take part.

If you decide to try a clinical trial, the trial you choose will depend on the type of cancer you have. It will also depend on the treatments you have already received. Each study has rules about who can take part. These rules may include the patient's age, health, and type of cancer. Clinical trials have both benefits and risks. Your doctor and the study doctors should tell you about these before you make any decisions.

Taking part in a clinical trial could help you and help others who get cancer in the future. But insurance and managed care plans do not always cover costs. What they cover varies by plan and by study. Talk with your health care team to learn more about coverage for clinical trials for your type of cancer.

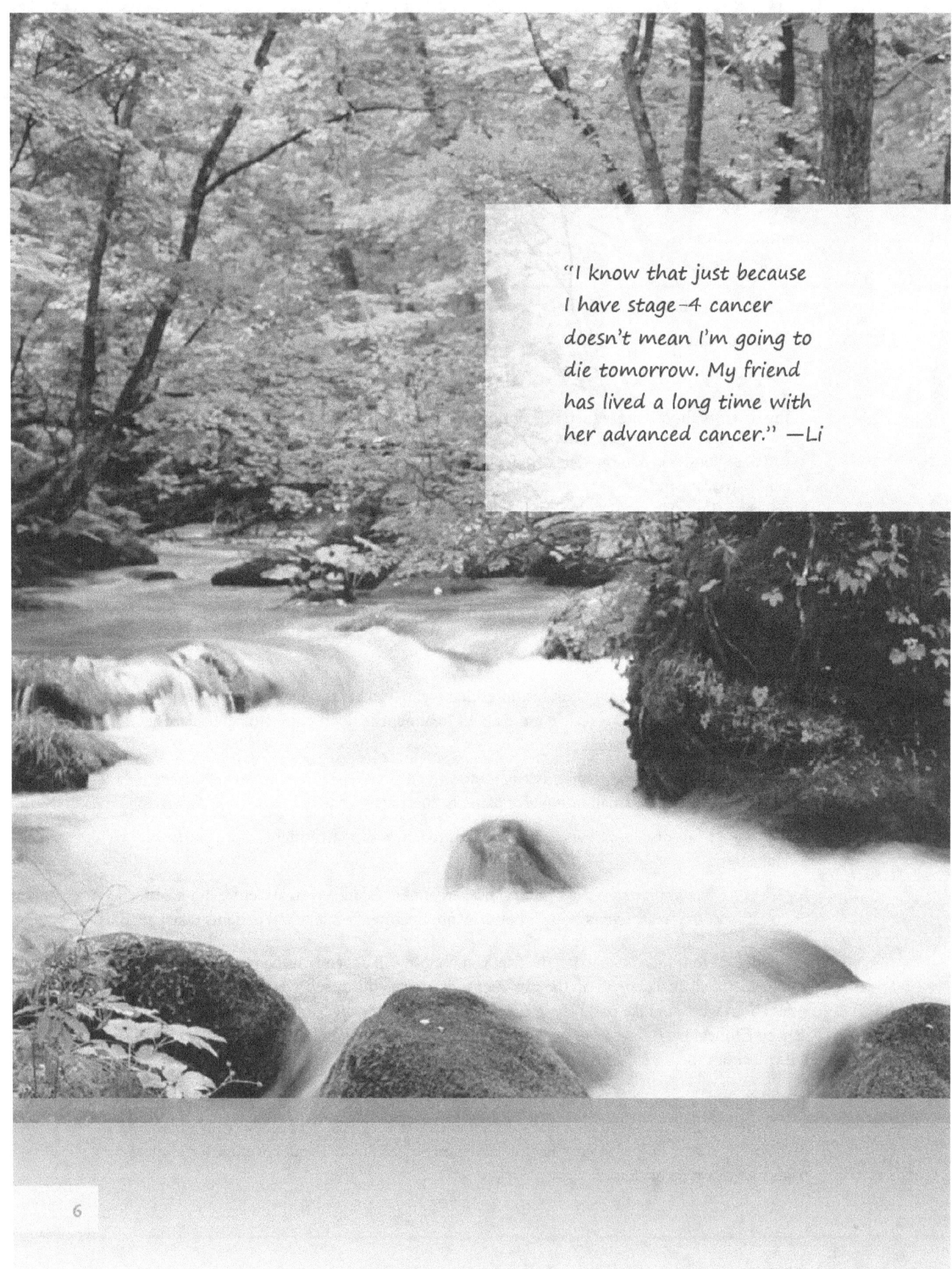

"I know that just because I have stage-4 cancer doesn't mean I'm going to die tomorrow. My friend has lived a long time with her advanced cancer." —Li

For more information about clinical trials, see NCI's booklet, *Taking Part in Cancer Treatment Research Studies.* Or talk to the NCI's Cancer Information Service at 1-800-422-6237 (1-800-4-CANCER).

Palliative Radiation, Chemotherapy, or Surgery

Some **palliative chemotherapy** and **palliative radiation** may help relieve pain and other symptoms. In this way, they may improve your quality of life, even if they don't stop your

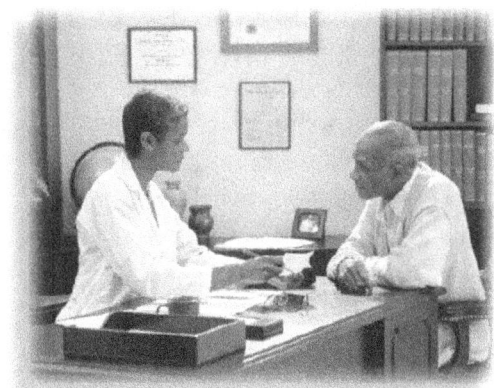

cancer. These treatments may be given to remove or shrink a **tumor.** Or they may be given to slow down a tumor's spread. **Palliative surgery** is sometimes used to relieve pain or other problems.

For more information, see the NCI booklets *Chemotherapy and You* and *Radiation Therapy and You.*

Hospice

Hospice care is an option if you feel you are no longer benefiting from cancer treatments. Choosing hospice care doesn't mean that you've given up. It just means the treatment goals are different at this point. It does not mean giving up hope, but rather changing what you hope for. But be sure to check with the hospice you use to learn what treatments and services are covered. Check with your insurance company also. The goal of hospice is to help patients live each day to the fullest by making them comfortable and lessen their symptoms. Hospice doctors, nurses, spiritual leaders, social workers, and volunteers are specially trained. They are dedicated to supporting their patients' and families' emotional, social, and spiritual needs, as well as dealing with patients' medical symptoms.

People usually qualify for hospice services when their doctor signs a statement that says that patients with their type and stage of disease, on average, aren't likely to survive beyond 6 months. Many people don't realize that they can use hospice services for a number of months, not just a few weeks. In fact, many say they wish they had gotten hospice care much sooner than they did. They were surprised by the expert care and understanding that they got. Often, control of symptoms not only improves quality of life but also helps people live longer. You will be reviewed periodically to see if hospice care is still right for you. Services may include:

- Doctor services (You may still keep your own doctors, too.)
- Nursing care
- Medical supplies and equipment
- Drugs to manage cancer-related symptoms and pain

Hospice and Home Care

What to Expect With Hospice Care

You can get hospice services at home, in special facilities, in hospitals, and in nursing homes. They have specialists to help guide care. They also have nurses on call 24 hours a day in case you need advice. And they have many volunteers who help families care for their loved one. Some hospices will give palliative chemotherapy at home as well. Hospice care doesn't seek to treat cancer, but it does treat reversible problems with brief hospital stays if needed. An example might be pneumonia or a bladder infection.

Medicare, Medicaid, and most private insurers cover hospice services. For those without coverage and in financial need, many hospices provide care for free. To learn more about hospice care, call the National Hospice and Palliative Care Organization at 1-800-658-8898. Or visit their website at http://www.nhpco.org. The website can also help you find a hospice in your community.

Benefits of Hospice and Home Care

Hospice and home care professionals can help you and your family work through some tough emotional issues. A social worker can offer emotional support, help in planning hospice or home care, and ease the move between types of care. Many people prefer the comfort of their own home, familiar surroundings, and having friends and family members nearby. Getting health care at home gives family members, friends, and neighbors the chance to spend time with you and help with your care.

- Short-term in-patient care
- Homemaker and home health aide services
- Respite (relief) services for caregivers. This means someone else helps with care for awhile, so the caregiver can take a break
- Counseling
- Social work services
- Spiritual care
- Bereavement (grief) counseling and support
- Volunteer services

Home Care

Home care services are for people who are at home rather than in a hospital. Home care services may include:

- Monitoring care
- Managing symptoms
- Providing medical equipment
- Physical and other therapies

You may have to pay for home care services yourself. Check with your insurance company. Medicare, Medicaid, and private insurance will sometimes cover home care services when ordered by your doctor. But some rules apply. So talk to your social worker and other members of your health care team to find out more.

CHAPTER 3

Talking With Your Health Care Team

As your disease advances, it's still important to give feedback to your doctor. That's the only way he or she can know what is working for you. Many people have a treatment team of health providers who work together to help them. This team may include doctors, nurses, **oncology social workers**, **dietitians**, and other **specialists**. They need to fully know your desires during treatment and at the end of your life. Let them know about any discomfort you have. You have a right to live your remaining days with dignity and peace of mind. So it's important to have a relationship and an understanding with those who will be caring for you.

Here are just a few topics you may want to discuss with your doctor or other members of your health care team:

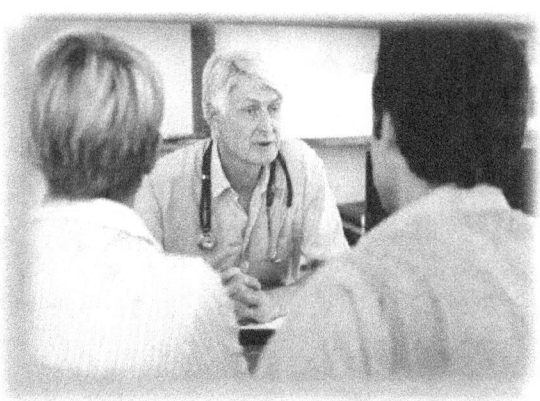

■ Pain or other symptoms. Be honest and open about how you feel. Tell your doctor if you have pain and where. Also tell him or her what you expect in the way of pain relief. (See Chapter 4 for more about pain and other symptoms.)

■ Communication. Some people want to know details about their care. Others prefer to know as little as possible. Some patients want their family members to make most of their decisions. What would you prefer? Decide what you want to know, how much you want to know, and when you've heard enough. Choose what is most comfortable for you, then tell your doctor and family members. Ask that they follow through with your wishes.

■ Family wishes. Some family members may have trouble dealing with cancer. They don't want to know how far the disease has advanced or how much time doctors think you have. Find out from your family members how much they want to know, and tell your health care team their wishes. Do this as soon as possible. It will help avoid conflicts or distress among your loved ones. (See Chapter 7 for more on talking to your loved ones.)

Remember that only you and those closest to you can answer many of these questions. Having answers to your questions can help you know what to expect now and in the future.

"My doctor said, 'The cancer is spreading to your lungs,' and from that moment on, I didn't hear a word he said. He started talking about my options, but all I saw were lips moving. I was in total shock." —Tyrone

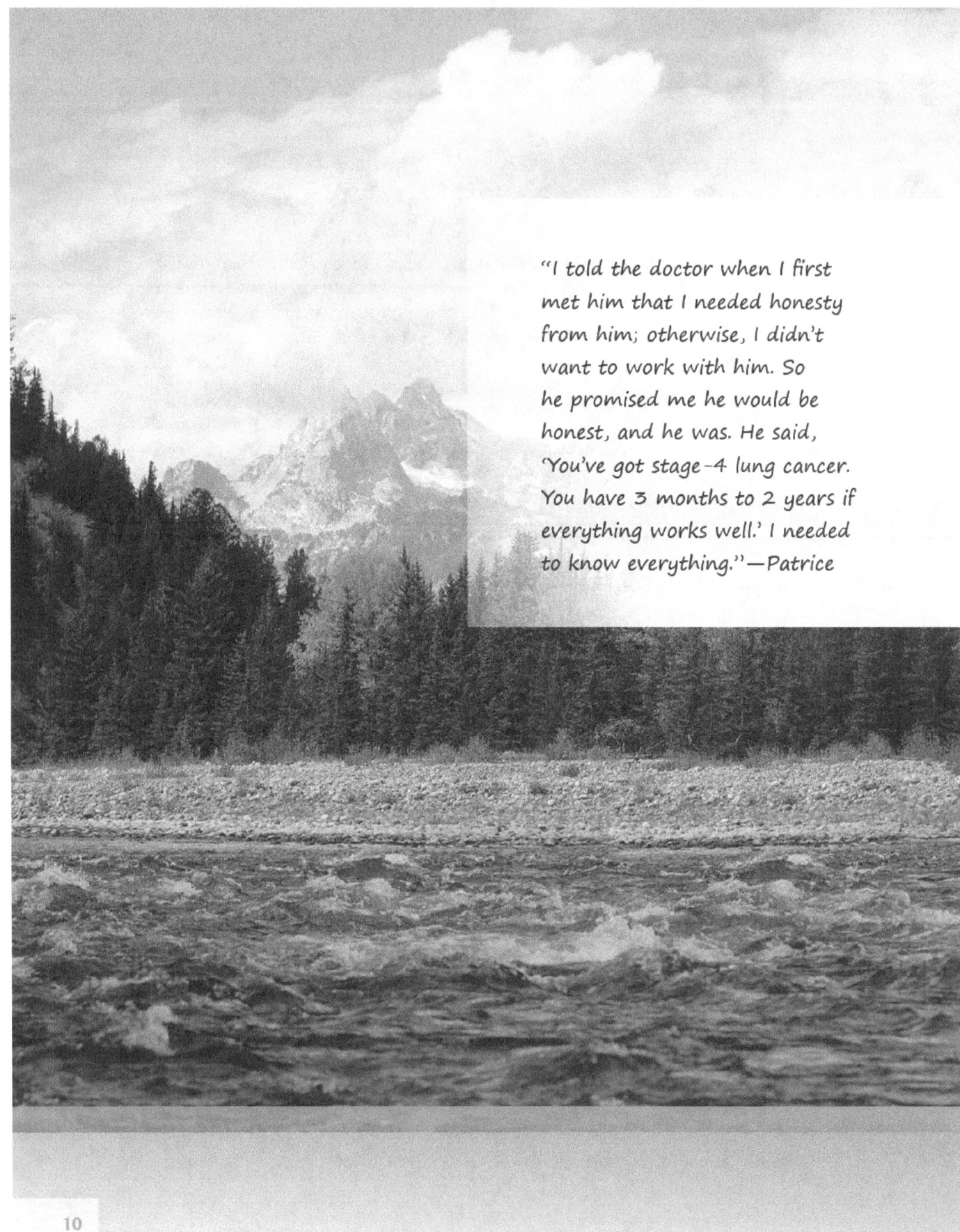

"I told the doctor when I first met him that I needed honesty from him; otherwise, I didn't want to work with him. So he promised me he would be honest, and he was. He said, 'You've got stage-4 lung cancer. You have 3 months to 2 years if everything works well.' I needed to know everything."—Patrice

Tips for Meeting With Your Health Care Team

■ Make a list of your questions before each appointment.

■ Bring a family member or trusted friend with you to your medical visits. This person can help you remember what the doctor or nurse said, and talk with you about it after the visit.

■ Ask all your questions. If you do not understand an answer, keep asking until you do. There is no such thing as a "stupid" question.

■ Take notes. You can do this or you can ask a family member or friend to take them for you. Or you can ask if it's okay to use a tape recorder.

■ Get a phone number of someone to call with follow-up questions.

■ Keep a file or notebook of all the papers and test results that your doctor has given you. Take this with you to your visits. Also keep records or a diary of all your visits. List the drugs and tests you have taken.

■ Keep a record of any upsetting symptoms or side effects you have. Note when and where they occur. Take this with you on your visits.

■ Find out what to do in an emergency. This includes whom to call, how to reach them, and where to go.

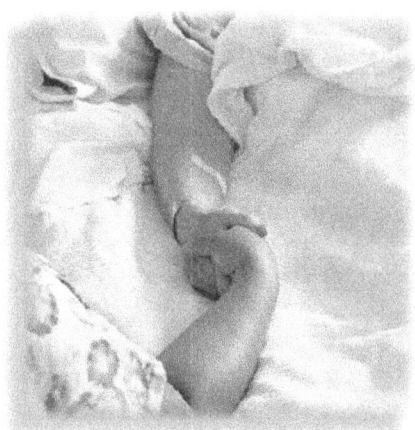

No One Knows the Future

It's normal for people to want to know how long they will have to live. It's also natural to want to prepare for what lies ahead. You may want to prepare emotionally as well as to make certain arrangements and plans.

But predicting how long someone will live is not exact. Your doctor may be able to give you an estimate, but keep in mind that it's a guess. Every patient is different. Your doctor has to take into account your type of cancer, treatment, past illnesses, and other factors.

Some patients live long past the time the doctor first predicted. Others live a shorter time. Also, an infection or other complication could happen and change things. Your doctor may know your situation best, but even he or she cannot know the answer for sure. And doctors don't always feel comfortable trying to give you an answer.

In truth, none of us knows when we are going to die. Unexpected events happen every day. The best we can do is try to live fully and for today.

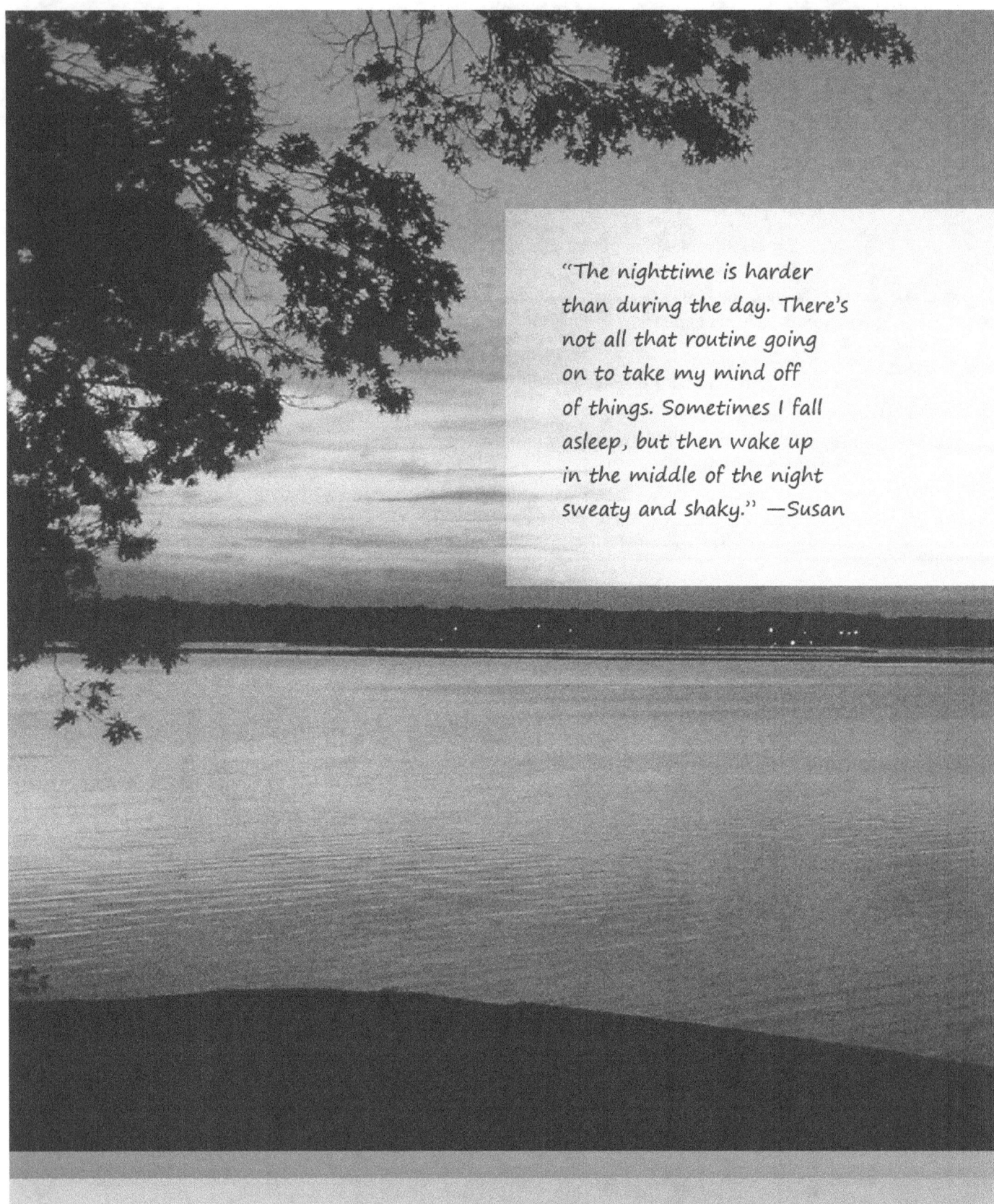

"The nighttime is harder than during the day. There's not all that routine going on to take my mind off of things. Sometimes I fall asleep, but then wake up in the middle of the night sweaty and shaky." —Susan

CHAPTER 4

Getting Help for Your Symptoms

Cancer and its treatment affect people differently. Some have symptoms, while others have no symptoms for a long time. As we said earlier, you have a right to comfort care throughout your illness.

Sometimes people assume their symptoms will get worse as their cancer progresses. But with good supports in place and good care, your symptoms should always be managed. So don't downplay your symptoms if you're having them. It's important to report how you are feeling. Tell your doctor, members of your health care team, and your loved ones. If you feel very sick or tired, your doctor may be able to adjust your treatment or give you other medicine.

Following are some of the symptoms you may have.

Pain

Having cancer doesn't always mean that you'll have pain. But if you do, you shouldn't accept pain as normal. Most types of pain can be treated. Your doctor can control pain with different medicines and treatments.

You may want to ask your doctor if you can talk to a pain specialist. Many hospitals have doctors on staff who are experts at treating pain. They may also have palliative medicine specialists.

Managing your pain helps you sleep and eat better. It makes it easier to enjoy your family and friends and focus on what gives you joy.

There are a few different ways to take pain medicine, including:

- By mouth
- Through the skin (like with a patch)
- By shots
- Through an **I.V.** or an **S.C.** pump

Your medicine, and how you take it, will depend on the type of pain and its cause. For example, for constant pain you may need a steady dose of medicine over a long period of time. You might use a patch placed on the skin or a slow-release pill.

Controlling Pain

What to Tell Your Doctor

When describing pain to your doctor, be as detailed as you can. Your doctor may ask:

- Where exactly is your pain? Does it move from one spot to another?

- How does the pain feel—dull, sharp, burning?

- How often does your pain occur?

- How long does it last?

- Does it start at a certain time— morning, afternoon, night?

- What makes the pain better? What makes it worse?

Using Strong Drugs To Control Pain

People with cancer often need strong medicine to help control their pain. Don't be afraid to ask for pain medicine or for larger doses if you need them. The drugs will help you stay as comfortable as you can be.

When treating pain in people with cancer, addiction is not an issue. Sadly, fears of addiction sometimes prevent people from taking medicine for pain. The same fears also prompt family members to encourage loved ones to "hold off" between doses. But people in pain get the most relief when they take their medicines and treatments on a regular schedule.

Medicines can be used for all types of pain, including:

- Mild to medium pain

- Medium to very bad pain

- **Breakthrough pain**

- Tingling and burning pain

- Pain caused by swelling

You should have regular talks with your healthcare team about the type and extent of your pain. That's because pain can change throughout your illness. Let them know the kind of pain you have, how bad it is, and where it hurts.

You may want to keep a "pain diary." Write down the information that's noted in the box on page 21. Include the time of day that the pain occurred and what you were doing. Rate the pain on a scale of 0 to 10. (Zero means no pain, and 10 is the worst pain you could have.) Use the diary when you talk to your doctor about your pain.

Unlike other medicines, there is no "right" dose for many pain medicines. Yours may be larger or smaller than someone else's. The right dose is the one that relieves your pain and makes you feel better.

Other Ways To Treat Pain

Cancer pain is usually treated with medicine and other therapies. But there are also some non-drug treatments. They are forms of **complementary and alternative medicine (CAM)**. Many people have found the methods listed below helpful. But talk with your health care team before trying any of them. Make sure they are safe and won't interfere with your cancer treatment.

- **Acupuncture** is a form of Chinese medicine that stimulates certain points on the body using small needles. It may help treat nausea and control pain. Before using acupuncture, ask your health care team if it is safe for your type of cancer.

- **Imagery** is imagining scenes, pictures, or experiences to feel calmer or perhaps to help the body heal.

- **Relaxation techniques** include deep breathing and exercises to relax your muscles.

- **Hypnosis** is a state of relaxed and focused attention. One focuses on a certain feeling, idea, or suggestion.

- **Biofeedback** is the use of a special machine to help the patient learn how to control certain body functions. These are things that we are normally not aware of (such as heart rate).

- **Massage therapy** brings relaxation and a sense of well-being by the gentle rubbing of different body parts or muscles. Before you try this, you need to check with your doctor. Massage is not recommended for some kinds of cancer.

These methods may also help manage stress. Again, talk to your health care team before using anything new, no matter how safe it may seem. Ask your health care team for more information about where to get these treatments. To learn more, see the NCI booklets *Thinking About Complementary and Alternative Medicine* and *Pain Control.*

Anxiety

Cancer takes a toll on both your body and your mind. You are coping with many different things now. You may feel overwhelmed. Pain and medicines for pain can also make you feel anxious or depressed. And you may be more likely to feel this way if you have had these feelings before.

Here are some signs of anxiety:

- Feeling very tense and nervous

- Racing heartbeat

- Sweating a lot

- Trouble breathing or catching your breath

- A lump in your throat or a knot in your stomach

- Sudden fear

Feeling anxious can be normal. But if it begins disrupting your daily life, ask for help from the members of your health care team. They can recommend someone for you to talk to. Counseling from a mental health professional has been shown to help many people cope with anxiety. Your doctor can also give you medicines that will help. Some of the complementary and alternative medicine choices listed above for pain may work for your anxiety as well. Art therapy and music therapy have also helped people cope.

Fatigue

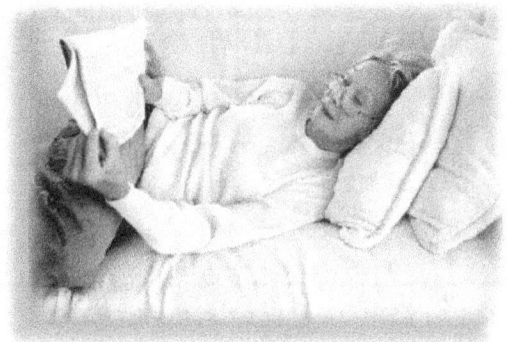

Fatigue is more than feeling tired. Fatigue is exhaustion—not being able to do even the small things you used to do. A number of things can cause fatigue. Besides cancer and its treatment, they include anxiety, stress, and changes in your diet or sleeping patterns. If you are having some of these problems, you might want to:

▓ Tell your health care team at your next visit. Some medicines can help with fatigue.

▓ Ask about your nutrition needs.

▓ Plan your daily activities. Do only what you really must do.

▓ Hand over tasks to others who are willing to help you.

▓ Include short periods of rest and relaxation every day.

▓ Take naps (no longer than 15-30 minutes).

▓ Ask others for help, especially when you are feeling fatigued.

▓ Do light exercises that are practical for you.

Nausea and Vomiting

Nausea and vomiting may be a problem for cancer patients. Both can make you feel very tired. They can also make it hard to get treatments or to care for yourself. If you feel sick to your stomach or are throwing up, there are many drugs to help you. Ask your health care team which medicines might work best for your nausea and vomiting.

You also may want to:

▓ Make small changes in your diet. Eat small amounts 5–6 times a day.

▓ Avoid foods that are sweet, fatty, salty, spicy, or have strong smells. These may make nausea and vomiting worse.

▓ Drink as much liquid as possible. You'll want to keep your body from getting dried out (dehydrated). Water, broth, juices, clear soft drinks, ice cream, and watermelon are good choices.

▓ Choose cool foods, which may help more than hot ones.

▓ Try acupuncture.

Constipation

Constipation is a problem in which stool becomes hard, dry, and difficult to pass, and bowel movements do not happen very often. Other symptoms may include painful bowel movements, and feeling bloated, uncomfortable, and sluggish. Chemotherapy, as well as other medicines (especially those used for pain), can cause constipation. It can also happen when people become less active and spend more time sitting or lying down.

Here are some ways to help manage constipation:

- Drink plenty of fluids each day. Many people find that drinking warm or hot fluids helps with bowel movements.

- Be active. You can be active by walking, doing water aerobics, or yoga. If you cannot walk, talk with your doctor or nurse about ways you can be active, such as doing exercises in bed or a chair.

- Ask your doctor, nurse, or dietitian if you should eat more fiber. He or she may suggest you eat bran, whole wheat bread and cereal, raw or cooked vegetables, fresh and dried fruit, nuts, and popcorn and other high-fiber foods.

- Let your doctor or nurse know if you are in pain or discomfort from not having a bowel movement. He or she may suggest you use an enema or take a laxative or stool softener. Check with your doctor or nurse before using any of these.

- Ask your doctor about giving you laxatives when you start to take pain medications. Taking a stool softener at the same time you start taking pain drugs may prevent the problem.

Loss of Appetite and Body Changes

Eating and appetite changes are common in the later stages of cancer. As your cancer progresses, your appetite may become poor.

On the other hand, you may be eating enough, but your body can't absorb the nutrients. This can cause you to lose weight, fat, and muscle.

Nutrition goals may become less important at this time. Even if your family members think you should have food, let your body be the judge. The goal should not be weight gain or improving your eating but rather comfort and symptom relief.

Your nurse, dietitian, and other members of your health care team can help. They can help you decide on changes to your diet that may be needed to keep you as healthy as possible. There are also new drugs to improve appetite and get rid of nausea. Ask your health care team about them.

Sleep Problems

Illness, pain, drugs, being in the hospital, and stress can cause sleep problems. Sleep problems may include:

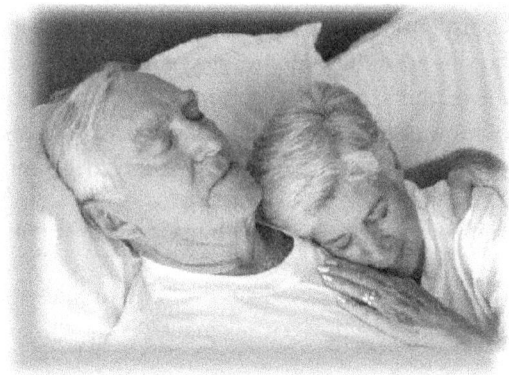

- Having trouble falling asleep
- Sleeping only in short amounts of time
- Waking up in the middle of the night
- Having trouble getting back to sleep

To help with your sleep problem, you may want to try:

- Reducing noise, dimming the lights, making the room warmer or cooler, and using pillows to support your body
- Dressing in soft, loose clothing
- Going to the bathroom before bed
- Eating a high-protein snack 2 hours before bedtime (such as peanut butter, cheese, nuts, or some sliced chicken or turkey)
- Avoiding caffeine (coffee, teas, colas, hot cocoa)
- Keeping regular sleep hours (avoid naps longer than 15-30 minutes)
- Talking with your health care team about drugs to help you sleep. These may give relief on a short-term basis.

Confusion

You may start noticing signs that you feel confused. This can occur in some people with advanced stage cancer. It can also be caused by some medicines. Confusion may begin suddenly or come and go during the day. Possible signs include:

- **Sudden changes in feelings** (such as feeling calm then suddenly becoming angry)
- **Having trouble paying attention or concentrating** (such as feeling easily distracted, having trouble answering questions, or finding it harder to do tasks that involve logic, such as math problems)
- **Memory and awareness problems** (such as forgetting where you are and what day it is or forgetting recent events)

If you notice these signs, talk to your health care team to try to find out the cause. Meanwhile, try one or more of the following to help relieve confusion:

- Go to a quiet, well-lit room with familiar objects.
- Reduce noise.
- Have family or loved ones nearby.
- Put a clock or calendar where it can be seen.
- Limit changes in caregivers.
- Ask your health care team about drugs that may help.

For more information on symptoms and side effects, see the NCI booklets:

- *Eating Hints*
- *Chemotherapy and You*
- *Radiation Therapy and You*
- *Pain Control*

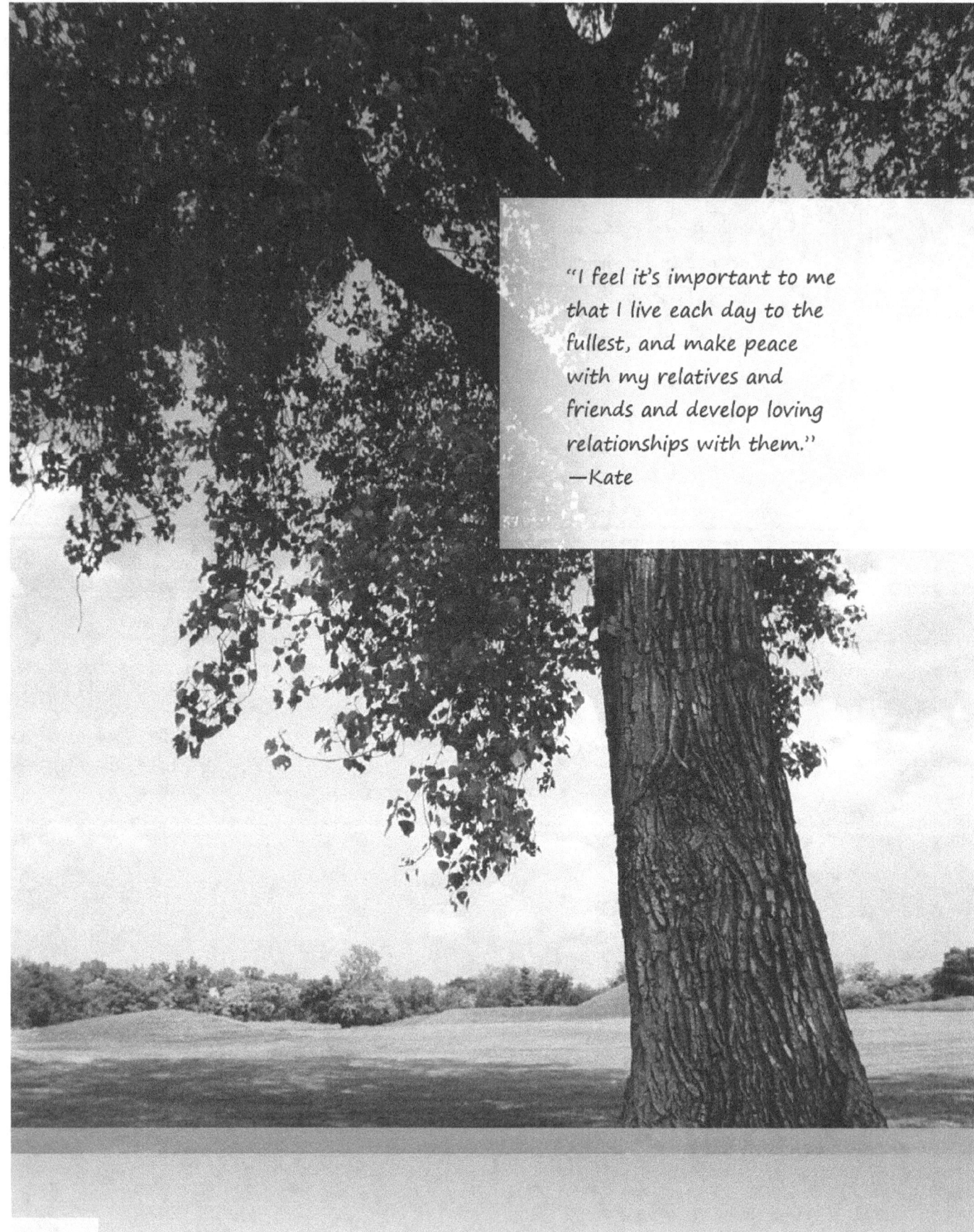

"I feel it's important to me that I live each day to the fullest, and make peace with my relatives and friends and develop loving relationships with them."
—Kate

CHAPTER 5

Coping With Your Feelings

You've probably felt a range of feelings during your cancer experience. You may have had these feelings at other times in your life, too, but they may be more intense now.

There is no right or wrong way to feel. And there is no right or wrong way to react to your feelings. Do what is most comfortable and useful for you.

You may relate to all of the feelings below or just a few. You may feel them at different times, with some days being better than others. It may help to know that others have felt the same way that you do. You may also want to read "Ways You Can Cope" on page 28. Some of the things others have done to cope with their feelings may help you, too.

Hope

You can feel a sense of hope, despite your cancer. But what you hope for changes with time. If you have been told that remission may not be possible, you can hope for other things. These may include comfort, peace, acceptance, even joy. Hoping may give you a sense of purpose. This, in itself, may help you feel better.

To build a sense of hope, set goals to look forward to each day. Plan something to get your mind off the cancer. Here are some tips from others with advanced stage cancer:

- Plan your days as you've always done.

- Don't stop doing the things you like to do just because you have cancer.

- Find small things in life to look forward to each day. You can also set dates and events to look forward to. Don't limit yourself. Look for reasons to hope, while staying aware of what's at hand.

Inner Strength

"My biggest struggle is that I need help, but I don't want people to give me too much of it. I want to do what I can for myself. If I have to work at something, there's a reason to live." —Will

People with cancer find strength they didn't know they had. You may have felt overwhelmed when you first learned that your doctors couldn't control your cancer. And now you aren't coping as well as you did in the past. But your feelings of helplessness may change. You may find physical and emotional reserves you didn't know you had. Calling on your inner strength can help revive your spirit.

Some people find it helpful to focus on the present instead of the past or future. They start a new daily routine. They accept that it may have to be different from the old routine. Others like to plan ahead and set goals. With places to go and things to do, life stretches out before them. Others focus on the relationships they have with people close to them. Inner strength is different for each person. So draw on the things in your life that are meaningful to you. Look at other sections in this booklet for ways to tap into your inner strength.

Sadness and Depression

It's normal to feel sad. You may have no energy or not want to eat. It's okay to cry or express your sadness in another way. You don't have to be upbeat all the time or pretend to be cheerful in front of others.

Pretending to feel okay when you don't doesn't help you feel better. And it may even create barriers between you and your loved ones. So don't hold it in. Do what feels natural to you.

Depression can happen if sadness or despair seems to take over your life. Some of the signs below are normal during a time like this. Talk to your doctor if they last for more than 2 weeks. Some symptoms could be due to physical problems. It's important to tell someone on your health care team about them.

Signs of Depression

- Feeling helpless or hopeless, or that life has no meaning

- Having no interest in family, friends, hobbies, or things you used to enjoy

- Losing your appetite

- Feeling short-tempered and grouchy

- Not being able to get certain thoughts out of your mind

- Crying for long periods of time or many times each day

- Thinking about hurting or killing yourself

- Feeling "wired," having racing thoughts or panic attacks

- Having sleep problems, such as not being able to sleep, having nightmares, or sleeping too much.

Your doctor can treat depression with medicine. He or she also may suggest that you talk about your feelings. You can do this with a psychologist or counselor. Or you may want to join a support group.

Grief

"I heard the doctor say, 'I'm so sorry, but . . .' and then I heard nothing else. My head was spinning, and I kept saying to myself, 'No, the doctor must be making a mistake.'" —Rosa

We all cope with loss or the threat of loss in different ways. You may feel sadness, loneliness, anger, fear, and guilt. Or you may find the way you think changes from time to time. For example, you may get easily confused or feel lost. Or your thoughts may repeat themselves over and over again. You may also find yourself low in energy. You may not want to do things or see people. These are all normal reactions to grief.

What you grieve for is as varied as how you think and feel. You may be grieving for the loss of your body as it used to be. You may grieve for the things you used to be able to do. You also may grieve losing what you have left: yourself, your family, your friends, your future. It's okay to take time for yourself and look inward. It's also okay to surround yourself with people who are close to you. Let your loved ones know if you want to talk. Let them know if you just want to sit quietly with them. There is no right or wrong way to grieve.

Often people who go through major change and loss need extra help. You can talk with a member of your health care team, a member of your faith community, or a mental health professional. You don't have to go through this alone.

Denial

"I feel like the reality of this cancer isn't going to go away if I deny it. If I did that, I might miss the comfort I get from sharing fears and concerns. I don't want to miss the sense of well-being I have knowing I have taken care of my loved ones." —Carrie

It's hard to accept the news that your cancer has spread or can no longer be controlled. And it's natural to need some time to adjust. But this can become a serious problem if it lasts longer than a few weeks. It can keep you from getting the care you need or talking about your treatment choices. As time passes, try to keep an open mind. Listen to what others around you suggest for your care.

Anger

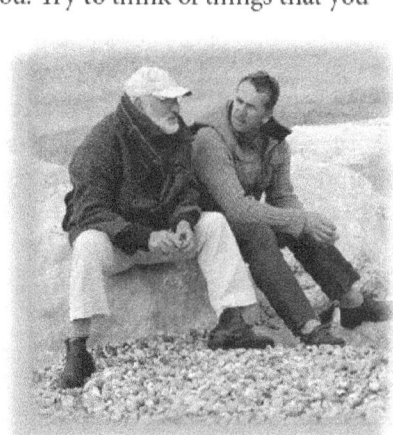

The feeling of "No, not me!" often changes to "Why me?" or "What's next?" You have a lot to deal with right now. It's normal and healthy to feel angry. You don't have to pretend that everything is okay. You may be mad at your doctor, family members, neighbors, and even yourself. Some people get angry with God and question their faith.

At first, anger can help by moving you to take action. You may decide to learn more about different treatment options. Or you may become more involved in the care you are getting. But anger doesn't help if you hold it in too long or take it out on others. Often the people closest to us are the ones who have to deal with our anger, whether we want that or not.

It may help to figure out why you are angry. This isn't always easy. Sometimes anger comes from feelings that are hard to show, such as fear, panic, worry, or helplessness. But being open and dealing with your anger may help you let go of it. Anger is also a form of energy. It may help to express this energy through exercise or physical activity, art, or even just hitting the bed with a pillow.

Stress

> "Just because I love God and know where I'm going, doesn't mean I'm not stressed. I worry all the time about what's to come. I try to focus on the things I can control, but it's not always easy." —David

Everyone has stress, but most likely you're having a lot more now. After all, you're dealing with many changes. Sometimes, you may not even notice that you're stressed. But your family and friends may see a change.

Anything that helps you feel calm or relaxed may help you. Try to think of things that you enjoy. Some people say it helps to:

- Exercise or take a walk.
- Write thoughts and feelings in a journal.
- Meditate, pray, or do relaxation exercises.
- Talk with someone about your stress.
- Do yoga or gentle stretching.
- Listen to soothing music.
- Express yourself through art.

Fear and Worry

"I have people around all day, but there's nothing worse than waking up alone and upset at 3:00 in the morning in a quiet, dark room. You have to have someone you can call right then." —Jamal

Facing the unknown is very hard. At times, you may feel scared of losing control of your life. You may be afraid of becoming dependent on other people. You may be afraid of dying.

If you struggle with these fears, remember that many others have felt the same way. Some people worry about what will happen to their loved ones in the future. Others worry about money. Many people fear being in pain or feeling sick. All these fears are normal.

Sometimes patients or family members worry that talking about their fears will make the cancer worse. This is not true. Thinking about getting sicker or dying is not going to make your health worse. But it's good to be hopeful and positive. It's better for your health to express your feelings, rather than hold them in.

Some people say it helps if you:

- **Know what to expect.** Learn more about your illness and treatment options by asking questions of your healthcare team.

- **Update your affairs.** If you have not already done so, make sure your will and other legal paperwork are in order. Then you won't have to worry about it. (See Chapter 6.)

- **Try to work through your feelings.** If you can, talk with someone you trust.

If you feel overwhelmed by fear, remember that others have felt this way, too. It's okay to ask for help.

Guilt and Regret

It's normal for people with cancer to wonder if they did anything to add to their situation. They may blame themselves for lifestyle choices. They may feel guilty because treatment didn't work. They may regret ignoring a symptom and waiting too long to go to the doctor. Others worry that they didn't follow the doctor's orders in the right way.

It's important to remember that the treatment failed you. You didn't fail the treatment. We can't know why cancer happens to some people and not others. In any case, feeling guilty won't help—it can even stop you from taking action and getting the treatment you need. So, it's important for you to:

- Try to let go of any mistakes you think you may have made.

- Focus on things worthy of your time and energy.

- Forgive yourself.

"I couldn't stop thinking about what I could have done to slow down my cancer. Maybe I should have gone to the doctor sooner, maybe I should have given up sweets, maybe I should have done this, maybe I should have done that. After talking about it with my social worker, she helped me see that this is no one's fault, especially mine." —Erika

You may want to share these feelings with your loved ones. Some people blame themselves for upsetting the people they love. Others worry that they'll be a burden on their families. If you feel this way too, take comfort in this: many family members have said it is an honor and a privilege to care for their loved one. Many consider it a time when they can share experiences and become closer to one another. Others say that caring for someone else makes them take life more seriously and causes them to rethink their priorities.

Maybe you feel that you can't talk openly about these things with your loved ones. If so, counseling or a support group may be an option for you. Let your health care team know if you would like to talk with someone.

Loneliness

> "I know my friends try to understand. It doesn't matter what I say though—they just don't get it. I can't even begin to explain to them how I feel or what's going on. I'm not saying it's their fault or anything. It's just hard." —Jennifer

You may feel alone, even if you have lots of people around you who care. You may feel that no one really understands what you're going through. And as the cancer progresses, you may see family, friends, or coworkers less often. You may find yourself alone more than you would like. Some people may even distance themselves from you because they have a hard time coping with your cancer. This can make you feel really alone.

Although some days may be harder than others, remember that you aren't alone. Keep doing the things you've always done the best you can. If you want to, tell people that you don't want to be alone. Let them know that you welcome their visits.

More than likely, your loved ones are feeling many of the same things you are. They, too, may feel cut off from you if they can't talk with you. You may also want to try joining a support group. There you can talk with others who share your feelings.

Finding Humor

Laughter can help you relax. Even a smile can fight off stressful thoughts. Of course, you may not always feel like laughing, but other people have found these ideas can help:

- Enjoy funny things children and pets do.

- Watch funny movies or TV shows.

- Read a joke book or look at jokes on the Internet. If you don't own a computer, use one at your local library. Or ask a friend to print some for you.

- Listen to comedy recordings.

- Read the comics in the newspaper or the cartoons and quotes in magazines.

- Look in the humor section in the library or book store.

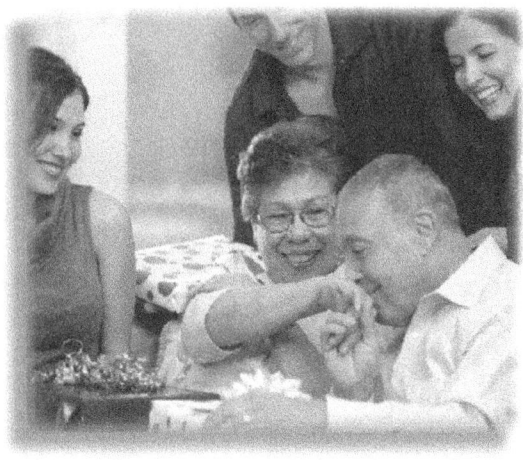

About Support Groups

You may have heard about support groups in your area for people with cancer. They can meet in person, by phone, or over the Internet. They may help you gain new insights into what's happening, get ideas about how to cope, and help you know that you're not alone.

In a support group, people may talk about their feelings and what they have gone through. They may trade advice and try to help others who are dealing with the same kinds of issues. Some people like to go and just listen. Others prefer not to join support groups at all. Some people aren't comfortable with this kind of sharing.

If you feel like you would enjoy outside support such as this, but can't get to a group in your area, try a support group on the Internet. Some people with cancer say that Websites with support groups have helped them a lot.

Getting Support

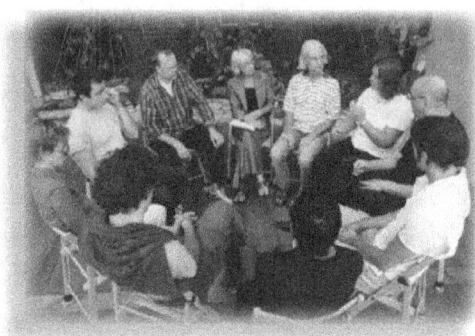

Your feelings will come and go, just as they always have in your life. It helps to have some strategies to deal with them.

First, know that you aren't alone. Many people have been in your situation. Some choose to confide in friends and family members. Others do better when they join a support group. It helps them to talk with others who are facing the same challenges. You may prefer to join an online support group, so you can chat with people from your home.

If support groups don't appeal to you, there are many experts who are trained to work in cancer care. These include oncology social workers, **health psychologists**, or counselors.

Many people also find faith as their source of support. They may seek comfort from the different members of their faith community. Or they may find that talking to a leader in their religious or spiritual community can be helpful. If you need help finding faith-based support, many hospitals have a staff chaplain who can give support to people of all faiths and religions. Your health care team may also be able to tell you about faith-based organizations in the area.

Ways You Can Cope

You may be able to keep doing many of your regular activities, even though some may be harder to do. Just remember to save your strength for the things you really want to do. Don't plan too many events for one day. Also, try to stagger things throughout the day.

On the next page you'll find some ideas that other patients say have helped them cope. As you can see, even little things can help.

Ways You Can Cope

Build model airplanes.

Pray or meditate.

Window shop.

People watch at the mall.

Go to a movie.

Play board games or cards.

Attend local concerts and plays.

Start a new daily routine. Accept that it may have to be different from your old one, but change is okay!

Talk about feelings with friends, family, or a leader in your spiritual or faith community.

Do yoga or gentle stretching.

I'm taking a watercolor class. I'm awful at it, but I sure don't care — anything that gets my mind off things.

I like to get my nails done.

I started to follow the stock market.

My nieces call and leave messages or songs on my answering machine. I listen to them when I need a fast way of cheering up.

Sometimes I drive out to the airport and watch planes. For some reason, it's very soothing to me.

I built a birdhouse with my grandson. We had fun, and I loved teaching him about tools.

I like to bird watch. I sit on my porch with a pair of binoculars.

I watch a lot of movies.

I like to fix things around the house.

I took up photography. I didn't buy a fancy camera or anything. I just started taking pictures.

Spend time outdoors in a community garden or park.

Volunteer or find a way to help others in need.

Plant flower pots.

Go to worship services.

Knit, crochet, or needlepoint.

Do crossword puzzles.

Do relaxation exercises.

Go fishing.

Do the things I enjoy, like making phone calls or reading.

Spend time with people I love.

Listen to music or a relaxation tape.

Do woodcarving.

Read mystery novels.

29

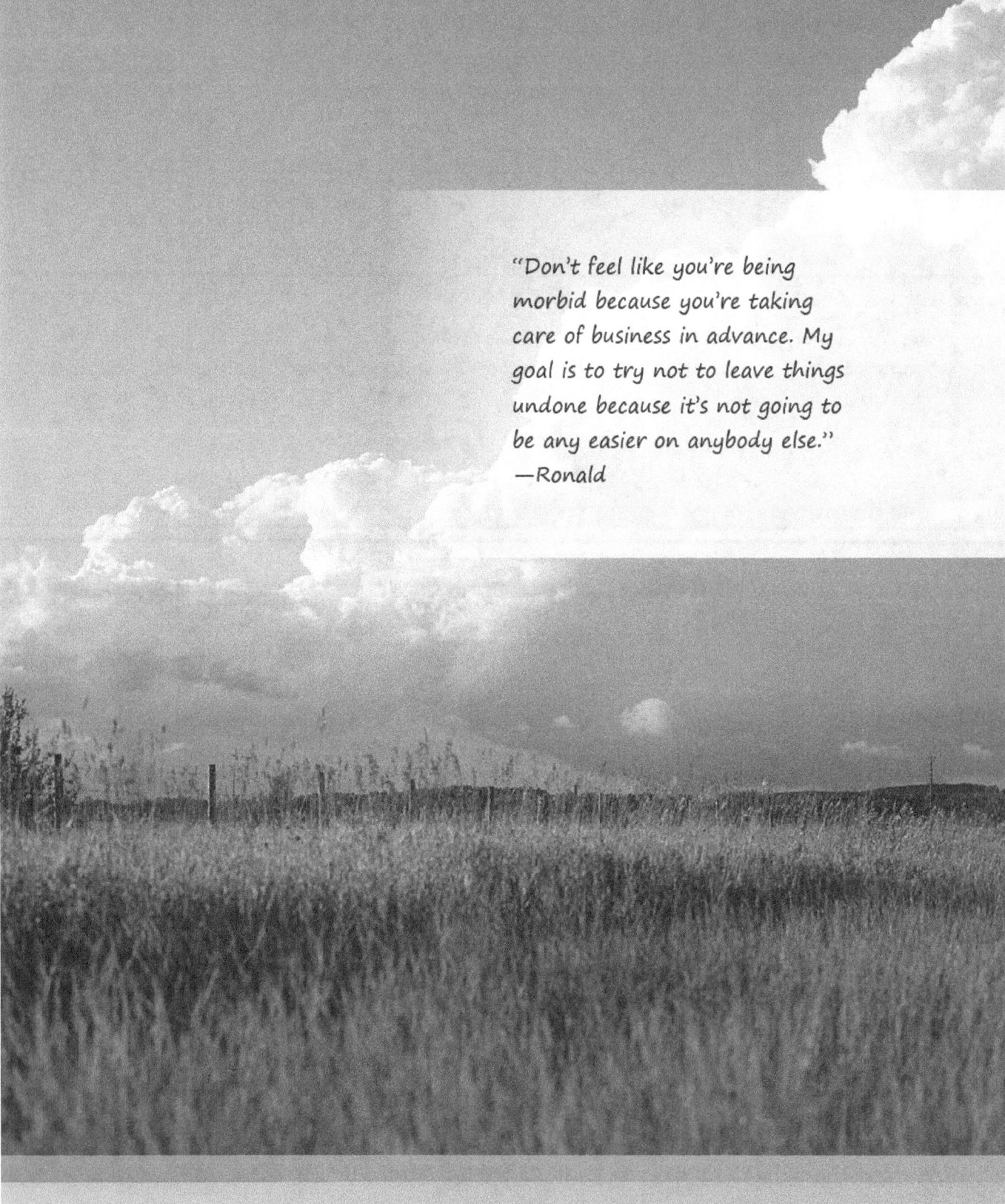

"Don't feel like you're being morbid because you're taking care of business in advance. My goal is to try not to leave things undone because it's not going to be any easier on anybody else."
—Ronald

CHAPTER 6

Advance Planning

This section outlines some things you can do to ensure your wishes are understood. This can help relieve the burden on your loved ones later.

Advance Directives

It's important to start talking about your wishes with the people who matter most to you. There may come a time when you can't tell your health care team what you need. Some people prefer to let their doctor or their family members make decisions for them. But often people with cancer feel better once they have made their desires known.

Advance directives are legal papers that tell your loved ones and doctors what to do if you can't tell them yourself. The papers let you decide ahead of time how you want to be treated. They may include a **living will** and a **durable power of attorney for health care**. Think about giving someone you trust the right to make medical decisions for you. This is one of the most important things you can do.

A living will lets people know what kind of medical care you want if you are terminally ill (dying). It states in writing your wishes about being kept alive by artificial means or extreme measures (such as a breathing machine or feeding tube). Some states allow you to give other instructions as well.

A durable power of attorney for health care names a person to make medical decisions for you when you can't make them yourself. (In some places, you can appoint this person to make decisions when you no longer want to.) This person is called a **health care proxy**. Choose a person you can trust to carry out your decisions and follow your preferences. Be sure to discuss this in-depth with the person you choose. They need to know they could be called upon. They should understand your wishes and any religious concerns you have.

Setting up an advance directive is not the same as giving up. Making decisions now keeps you in control. You are making your wishes known for all to follow. This can help you worry less about the future and live each day to the fullest.

It's hard to talk about these issues. But it often comforts family members to know what you want. And it saves them having to bring up the subject themselves. You may also gain peace of mind. You are making hard choices for yourself instead of leaving them to your loved ones.

Make copies of your advance directives. Give them to your family members, your health care team, and your hospital medical records department. This will ensure that everyone knows your decisions.

Following State Laws

You do not always need a lawyer present to fill out these documents. But you may need a notary public. Each state has its own laws concerning living wills and durable powers of attorney. These laws can vary in important details. In some states, a living will or durable power of attorney signed in another state isn't legal. Talk with your lawyer or social worker to get more details.

Or look at your state's government website. (See the Resources section at the end of the booklet for more on how to get copies of advance directives.)

Other Legal Papers

Here are some other legal papers that are not part of the advance directives:

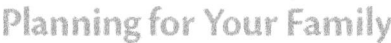

- A **will** divides your property among your heirs.

- A **trust** is when a person you appoint oversees, invests, or pays out money to those named in the trust.

- **Legal power of attorney**—you appoint a person to make financial decisions for you when you can't make them yourself.

Planning for Your Family

Careful planning reduces the financial, legal, and emotional burden your family and friends will face after you're gone. For many people, it's hard bringing up these subjects. But talking about them now can avoid problems later.

Maybe you don't feel comfortable bringing up the subject with loved ones. Or maybe your family simply doesn't talk about these things. In either case, seek help from a member of your health care team. They may be able to help your family understand.

- **Clearing up insurance issues.** Contact your health insurance company if you decide to try a new treatment or go into hospice. Most insurance plans cover hospice. They also cover brief home visits from a nurse or a home health aide several times a week. But it's wise to ask in advance. This may prevent payment problems later.

- **Putting your affairs in order.** You can help your family by organizing records, insurance policies, documents, and instructions. You may want to call your bank to make sure you have taken all the right steps in doing these things. On the next page is a checklist to share with the person who will help you manage your affairs. (Also see the Personal Affairs Worksheet on page 50.)

- **Making funeral arrangements.** You may want to help your family plan a funeral or memorial service that has your personal touch. Some people plan services that are celebrations. Talk with your family about how you want others to remember you.

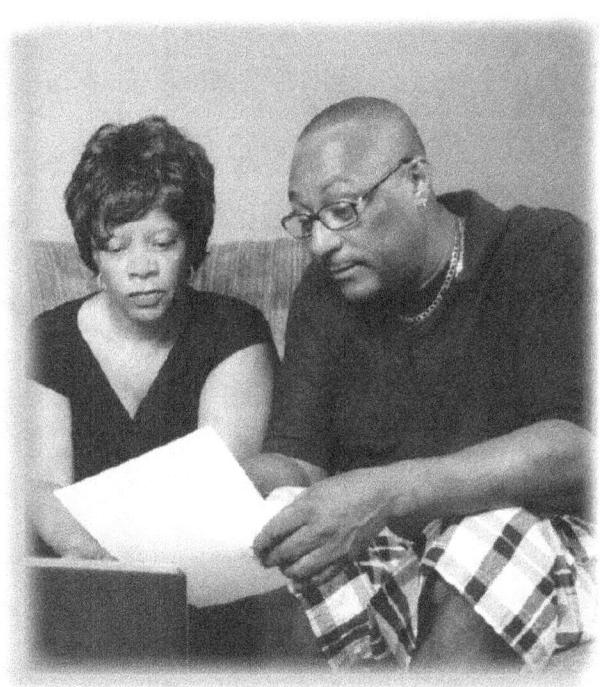

A Checklist for Organizing Your Affairs

✔ If you can't physically gather important papers, make a list of where your family can find them.

✔ Keep your papers in a fireproof box or with your lawyer.

✔ If you keep your important papers in a safety deposit box, make sure that a family member or friend has access to the box.

✔ Although original documents are needed for legal purposes, give family members photocopies.

A worksheet of important papers and documents is on page 50. You can use it as a guide to the types of papers your family will need.

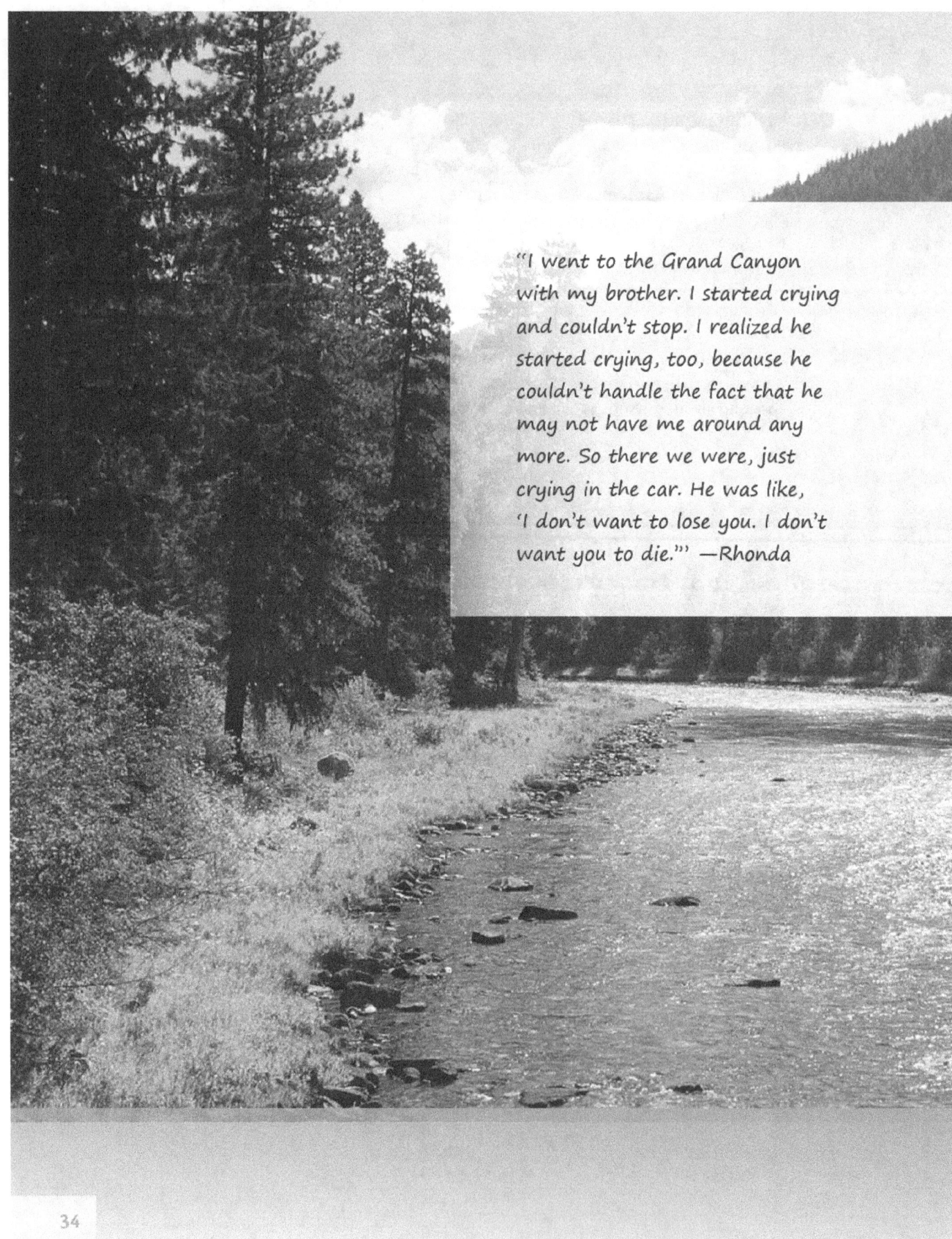

"I went to the Grand Canyon with my brother. I started crying and couldn't stop. I realized he started crying, too, because he couldn't handle the fact that he may not have me around any more. So there we were, just crying in the car. He was like, 'I don't want to lose you. I don't want you to die.'" —Rhonda

CHAPTER 7

Talking With the Special People in Your Life

Your loved ones may need time to adjust to the new stage of your illness. They need to come to terms with their own feelings. These may include confusion, shock, helplessness, or anger. Let them know that they can offer comfort just by being themselves and by being at ease with you. Ask them to listen when you need it, rather than try to solve every problem.

Knowing that people cope with bad news in their own way will help you and your loved ones deal with their emotions. Many people are reassured and comforted by sharing feelings and taking the time to say what they need to.

Bear in mind that not everyone can handle the thought that they might lose you. Or some people may not know what to say or do for you. As a result, relationships may change. This isn't because of you, but because others have trouble coping with their own painful feelings.

If you can, remind them that you are still the same person you always were. Let them know if it's all right to ask questions or tell you how they feel. Sometimes just reminding them to be there for you is enough. But it's also okay if you don't feel comfortable talking about it either. Sometimes certain topics are hard to talk about with others. If this is the case, you may want to talk by yourself with a member of your medical team or a trained counselor. You also may want to attend a support group where people meet to share common concerns.

Some families have trouble expressing their needs to each other. Other families simply do not get along with each other.

If you don't feel comfortable talking with family members, ask a member of your health care team to help. You could also ask a social worker or other professional to hold a family meeting. This may help family members feel safer to express their feelings openly. It can also be a time for you and your family to meet with your team to problem-solve and set goals.

It can be very hard to talk about these things. But studies show that cancer care goes more smoothly when everyone stays open and talks about the issues.

Often, talking with the people closest to you is harder than talking with anyone else. Here's some advice on talking with loved ones during tough times.

Spouses and Partners

Some relationships grow stronger during cancer treatment, but others are weakened. It's very common for patients and their partners to feel more stress than usual as a couple. There is often stress about:

- Knowing how to give and get support

- Coping with new feelings that have come up

- Figuring out how to communicate

- Having money problems

- Making decisions

- Changing roles

- Having changes in social life

- Coping with changes in daily routines

Some people feel more comfortable talking about serious issues than others. Only you and your loved one know how you communicate. Some things to think about are:

- **Talk things over.** This may be hard for you or your partner. If so, ask a counselor or social worker to talk to both of you together.

- **Be realistic about demands.** Your spouse or partner may feel guilty about your illness. They may feel guilty about any time spent away from you. They also may be under stress due to changing family roles.

- **Spend some time apart.** Your partner needs time to address his or her own needs. If these needs are neglected, your loved one may have less energy and support to give. Remember, you didn't spend 24 hours a day together before you got sick.

- **Know that it's normal for body changes and emotional concerns to affect your sex life.** Talking openly and honestly is key. But if you can't talk about these issues, you might want to talk with a professional. Don't be afraid to seek help or advice if you need it.

"My wife has been my biggest source of strength, plain and simple. That's how I cope with all of it, because we talk and sometimes we literally are talking until 4 or 5 in the morning. We are just sitting here and just talking and reminiscing, and asking questions and answering them. Being there for one another." —Steve

Small Children

"We can't always protect the people we love. But we can prepare them."
—Unknown

Keeping your children's and grandchildren's trust is still very important at this time. Children can sense when things are wrong. It's best to be as open as you can about your cancer. They may worry that they did something to cause the cancer. They may be afraid that no one will take care of them. They may also feel that you are not spending as much time with them as you used to. Although you can't protect them from what they may feel, you can prepare them.

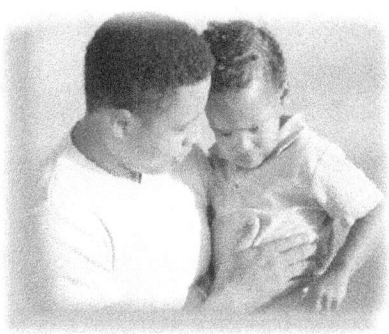

Some children become very clingy. Others get into trouble in school or at home. Let the teacher or guidance counselor know what is going on. And with your kids, it helps to keep the lines of communication open. Try to:

- Be honest. Tell them you are sick and that the doctors are working to help you feel comfortable.

- Let them know that nothing they did or said caused the cancer. And make sure they know that they can't catch it from others.

- Tell them you love them.

- Tell them it's okay to be upset, angry, or scared. Encourage them to talk.

- Be clear and simple, since children do not have the focus of adults. Use words they can understand.

- Let them know that they will be taken care of and loved.

- Let them know that it's okay to ask questions. Tell them you will answer them as honestly as you can. In fact, children who aren't told the truth about an illness can become even more scared. They often use their imagination and fears to explain the changes around them.

Teenagers

"My father and I are so much closer. It's a totally different family than we were before I was diagnosed. We've learned how to talk about how we feel, how to talk to each other about what's going on and what we're afraid of."
—Jake

Many of the things listed above also apply to teenagers. They need to hear the truth about an illness. This helps keep them from feeling guilt and stress. But be aware that they may try to avoid the subject. They may become angry, act out, or get into trouble as a way of coping. Others simply withdraw. Try to:

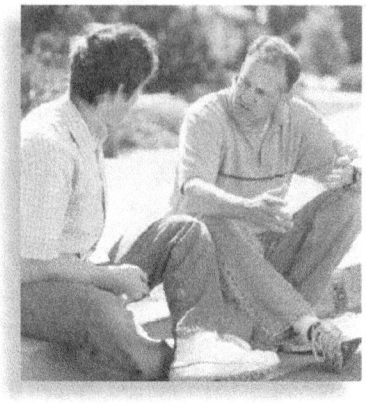

- Give teenagers the space they need. This is especially important if you rely on them more than before to help with family needs.

- Give them time to deal with their feelings, alone or with friends.

- Let your teenager know that they should still go to school and take part in sports and other fun activities.

If you have trouble explaining your illness, you might want to ask for help. Try asking a close friend, relative, or health care provider for advice. You could also go to a trusted coach, teacher, or youth minister. Your social worker or doctor can help you find a good counselor.

Adult Children

Your relationship with your adult children may change now that you have advanced cancer. You may have to rely on them more for different needs. It may be hard for you to ask for support. After all, you may be used to giving support rather than getting it. Or it may be hard for other reasons; perhaps your relationship with them has been distant.

Adult children have their concerns, too. They may become fearful of their own mortality. They may feel guilty because they feel that they can't meet the many demands on their lives as parents, children, and employees.

As your illness progresses, it helps to:

- Share decision-making with your children.

- Involve them in issues that are important to you. These may include treatment choices, plans for the future, or types of activities you want to continue.

Reaching out to your children and openly sharing your feelings, goals, and wishes may help them cope with your disease. It may also help lessen fears and conflict between siblings when other important decisions need to be made.

"It's a roller coaster ride, so we just ride the roller coaster. I've got the whole family prepared, and that's what you have to do when you have cancer. Things are going well and then really bad." —Delia

CHAPTER 8

Looking for Meaning

Many people who have advanced cancer look more deeply for meaning in their lives. They want to understand their purpose and their legacy. They want to examine the things they have gone through in life. Some look for a sense of peace or a bond with others. Some seek to forgive themselves or others for past actions. Some look for answers and strength through religion or spirituality.

Being spiritual can mean different things to different people. It can be a very personal issue. Everyone has their own beliefs about the meaning of life. Some people find it through religion or faith. Some people find it by teaching, or through volunteer work. Others find it in different ways. Having cancer may cause you to think about what you believe. You may think about God, an afterlife, about the connections made between living things. This can bring a sense of peace, a lot of questions, or both.

Like some people, you may also find that cancer changes your values. Having the disease may help you learn what is most important to you. The things you own and your daily duties may seem less important. You may decide to spend more time with loved ones or helping others. You may want to do more things in the outdoors, or learn something new.

You may have already given a lot of thought to these issues. Still, you might find comfort by exploring more deeply what is meaningful to you. You could do this with someone close to you, a member of your faith community, or a mental health professional.

Or you may just want to take time for yourself. You may want to reflect on your experiences and relationships. Writing in a journal or reading also helps some people find comfort and meaning. Many people find that prayer, meditation, or talking with others has helped them cope and explore their lives.

Celebrating Your Life

Having advanced cancer often gives people a chance to look back on life and all they have done. They like to look at the different roles they have played throughout life. They think about what something meant at the time, and what it means now. Some gather things that have meaning to them to give to their loved ones. Others share memories or projects with loved ones.

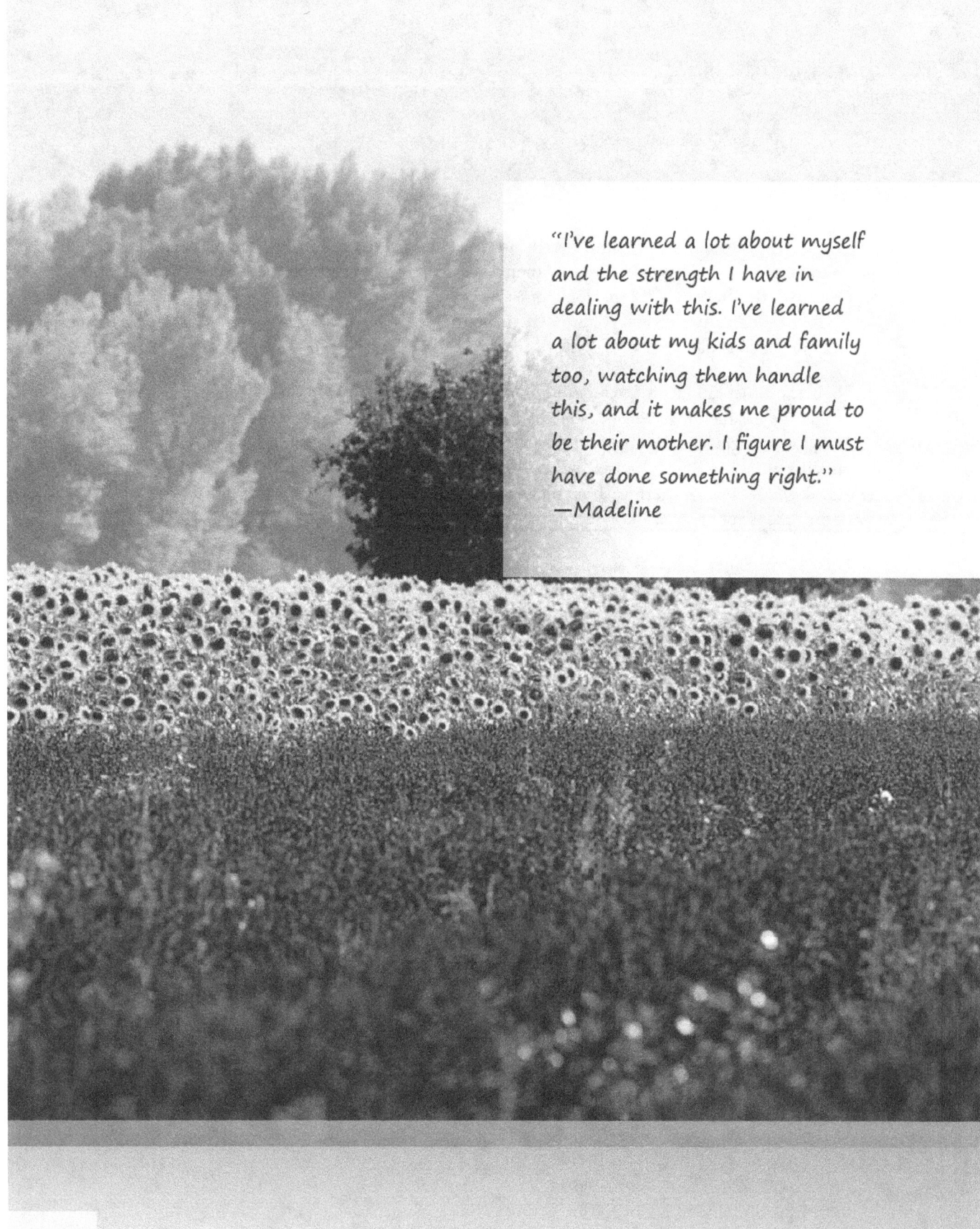

"I've learned a lot about myself and the strength I have in dealing with this. I've learned a lot about my kids and family too, watching them handle this, and it makes me proud to be their mother. I figure I must have done something right."
—Madeline

Doing these things is often called "making a legacy" for yourself. It can be whatever you want. Don't limit yourself! And you can do these things alone or with others close to you. Some examples of ways people have celebrated their lives are:

- Making a video of special memories

- Reviewing or arranging family photo albums

- Charting or writing down your family's history or family tree

- Keeping a daily journal of your feelings and experiences

- Making a scrapbook

- Writing notes or letters to loved ones and children

- Reading or writing poetry

- Creating artwork, knitting, or making jewelry

- Giving meaningful objects or mementos to loved ones

- Writing down or recording funny or special stories from your past

- Planting a garden

- Making a recording of favorite songs

- Gathering favorite recipes into a cookbook

You can do whatever you want that brings joy and meaning to you. Some people with cancer also make what is called an "**ethical will.**" It's not a legal paper. It's something you write yourself to share with your loved ones. Many ethical wills contain the person's thoughts on his or her values, memories, and hopes. They may also talk about the lessons learned in life or other things that are meaningful. It can say anything you want, in any way you want.

"For the meaning of life differs from man to man, from day to day and from hour to hour. What matters, therefore, is not the meaning of life in general but rather the specific meaning of a person's life at a given moment." —Viktor Frankl

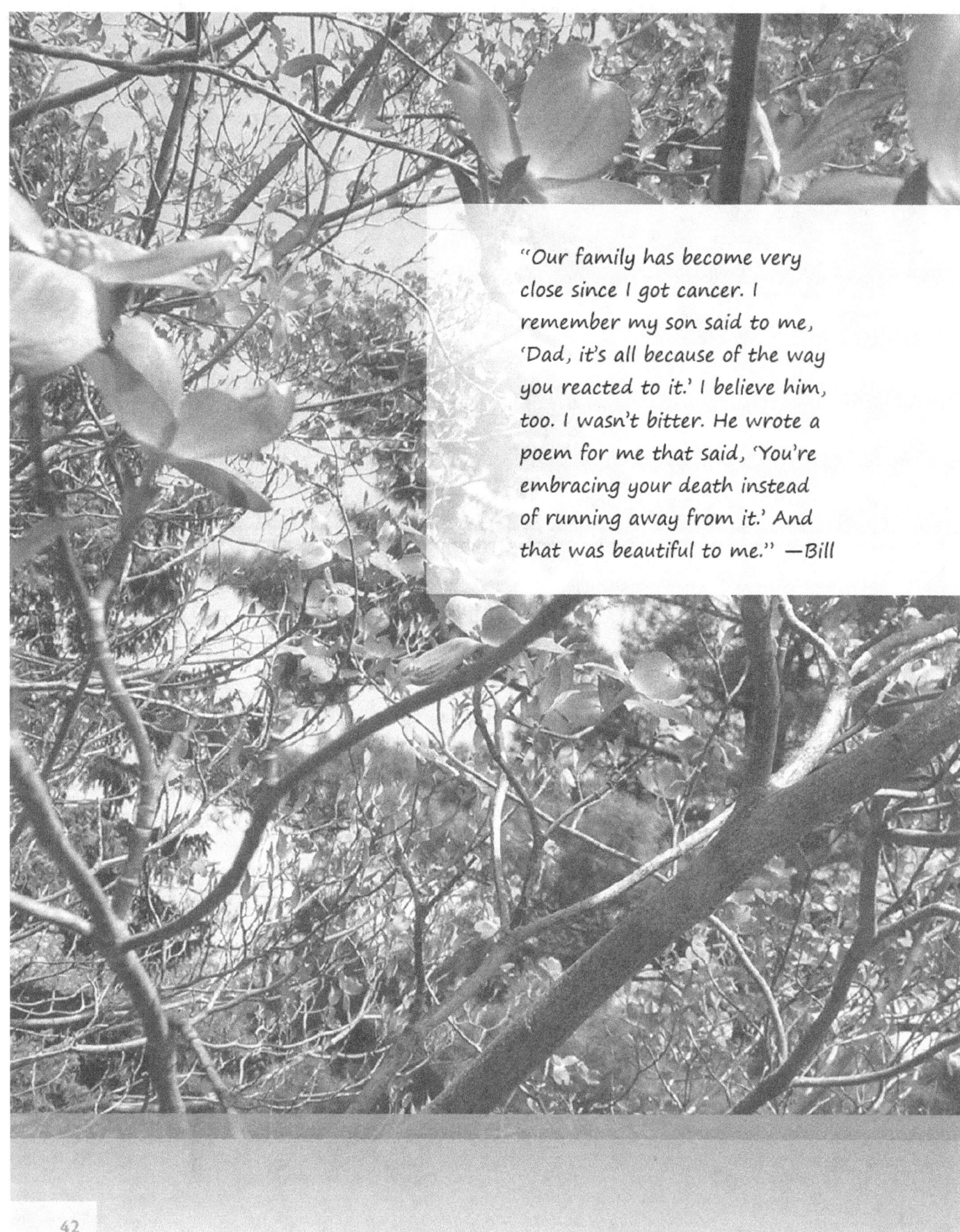

"Our family has become very close since I got cancer. I remember my son said to me, 'Dad, it's all because of the way you reacted to it.' I believe him, too. I wasn't bitter. He wrote a poem for me that said, 'You're embracing your death instead of running away from it.' And that was beautiful to me." —Bill

CHAPTER 10

Closing Thoughts

Living with advanced stage cancer may bring many challenges and hardships. But it can also be a time of fulfillment and joy.

As you think about the issues raised in this booklet, keep in mind that survival statistics are just numbers. The numbers that really mean the most for any of us are quite different. They measure the good days, the comfortable nights, and the hours of happiness and joy. Keep living your life the best that you can and in the fullest way possible.

"Think only of today, and when tomorrow comes, it will be today, and we will think about it." —St. Francis de Sales

Resources

Cancer Information and Support

Federal Resources

For more resources:

See *National Organizations That Offer Cancer-Related Services* at http://www.cancer.gov. In the search box, type in the words "national organizations."

Or call 1-800-4-CANCER (1-800-422-6237) to seek more help.

■ National Cancer Institute

Provides current information on cancer prevention, screening, diagnosis, treatment, clinical trials, genetics, and supportive care.

Visit......................http://www.cancer.gov

■ Cancer Information Service

Answers questions about cancer, clinical trials, and cancer-related services and helps users find information on the NCI website. Provides NCI printed materials.

Toll-free......................1-800-4-CANCER (1-800-422-6237)

Visit...............................http://www.cancer.gov/aboutnci/cis

Chat online...............Click on "LiveHelp" online chat from the home page.

■ Administration on Aging

Provides information, assistance, individual counseling, organization of support groups, caregiver training, respite care, and supplemental services.

Phone...................1-202-619-0724

Visit......................http://www.aoa.gov

■ Centers for Medicare and Medicaid Services

Provides information for consumers about patient rights, prescription drugs, and health insurance issues, including Medicare and Medicaid.

Toll-free 1-800-MEDICARE (1-800-633-4227)

Visit......................http://www.medicare.gov (for Medicare information) or
http://www.cms.hhs.gov (other information)

■ Equal Employment Opportunity Commission

Provides fact sheets about job discrimination, protections under the Americans With Disabilities Act, and employer responsibilities. Coordinates investigations of employment discrimination.

Toll-free 1-800-669-4000

TTY 1-800-669-6820

Visit......................http://www.eeoc.gov

U.S. Department of Labor Office of Disability Employment Policy

Provides fact sheets on a variety of disability issues, including discrimination, workplace accommodation, and legal rights.

Toll-free 1-866-633-7365

TTY 1-877-889-5627

Visit ....http://www.dol.gov/odep

Private/NonProfit Organizations

Aging With Dignity

Provides information and materials regarding advance directives. You can order the document Five Wishes, which states your end of life decisions for your health care team, and friends and family members.

Toll-free 1-888-5WISHES (1-888-594-7437)

Visit ....http://www.agingwithdignity.org

American Cancer Society National Cancer Information Center

Available to answer questions 24 hours a day, 7 days a week.

Toll-free 1-800-ACS-2345 (1-800-227-2345)

Visit ....http://www.cancer.org

CancerCare

Offers free support, information, financial assistance, and practical help to people with cancer and their loved ones.

Toll-free 1-800-813-HOPE (1-800-813-4673)

Visit ....http://www.cancercare.org

Cancer Support Community

The CSC is dedicated to providing support, education, and hope to people affected by cancer.

Toll-free 1-888-793-9355

Visit ....http://www.cancersupportcommunity.org

Hospice Foundation of America

Provides programs and materials on hospice care, caregiving, grief, and end of life. They also provide a hospice locator service, and links to other organizations and resources.

Toll-free 1-800-854-3402

Visit ....http://www.hospicefoundation.org

■ **Kids Konnected**

Offers education and support for children who have a parent with cancer or who have lost a parent to cancer.

Toll-free 1-800-899-2866

Visit .... http://www.kidskonnected.org

■ **National Coalition for Cancer Survivorship**

Provides information on cancer support, employment, financial and legal issues, advocacy, and related issues.

Toll-free: .... 1-877-NCCS YES (1-877-622-7937)

Visit .... http://www.canceradvocacy.org

■ **National Hospice and Palliative Care Organization**

Provides information on hospice care, local hospice programs, state specific advance directives, and locating a local health care provider. Through their program, Caring Connections, they also provide education and materials on palliative and end of life issues, as well as links to other organizations and resources.

Toll-free 1-800-658-8898

Visit .... http://www.nhpco.org

■ **Caring Connections**

Toll-free 1-800-658-8898

Visit .... http://www.caringinfo.org

■ **NeedyMeds—Indigent Patient Programs**

Lists medicine assistance programs available from drug companies.
NOTE: Usually patients cannot apply directly to these programs. Ask your doctor, nurse, or social worker to contact them.

Visit .... http://www.needymeds.com

■ **Patient Advocate Foundation**

Offers education, legal counseling, and referrals concerning managed care, insurance, financial issues, job discrimination, and debt crisis matters.

Toll-free 1-800-532-5274

Visit .... http://www.patientadvocate.org

Words to Know

Acupuncture (AK-yoo-PUNK-cher): A form of Chinese medicine that stimulates certain points on the body. The goal is to promote health. It is also used to lessen disease symptoms and treatment side effects. For people with cancer, it may help treat nausea and control pain. Before using acupuncture, ask your health care team if it is safe for your type of cancer.

Advance directives: Legal papers that allow you to decide ahead of time how you want to be treated when you are dying. The two main types are living wills and durable power of attorney.

Advanced cancer: Cancer that doctors no longer believe they can control with treatment; also called "advanced stage cancer" or "late-stage cancer."

Biofeedback: A way to monitor certain body functions to gain some control over them. Examples of such body functions are heart rate and blood pressure.

Breakthrough pain: Pain that "breaks through" pain medication or is very painful for a short time. Breakthrough pain can occur several times a day. This can happen even when a patient is taking the right dose of pain control medicine.

Complementary and alternative medicine (CAM): Treatment used along with, or instead of, standard health care. CAM includes methods such as acupuncture and massage. Some CAM treatments may help relieve cancer symptoms or side effects. But not all CAM treatments are safe. They should not take the place of standard health care.

Clinical trials: A type of research study that uses volunteers to test new methods of screening, prevention, diagnosis, or treatment of a disease. Also called a clinical study.

Diagnosis (dye-ug-NOH-sis): The name and details of your disease or health condition. In recurrent cancer, this includes your type, location, and stage of cancer.

Dietitian (dy-uh-TIH-sun): A person with special training in nutrition, who can help you with choices in your diet. They also can suggest ways to make eating easier.

Durable power of attorney for health care: This type of advance directive appoints a person (healthcare proxy). The healthcare proxy makes health care decisions for you when you can't make them yourself.

Ethical (EH-thuh-kul) will: A paper that contains thoughts or wishes that you want to share with your loved ones. An ethical will is not a legal document.

Health psychologist: A mental health professional who works with people and families affected by illness.

Health care proxy: The person you have named in an advance directive to make medical decisions for you. This person can make choices for your care when you can't make them yourself.

Hospice (HA-spis) **care**: Care given to help patients live each day to the fullest and die with dignity. The goal of hospice care is not to treat the disease but to make the patient comfortable and symptom free.

Hypnosis: A state of relaxed and focused attention. The patient focuses on a certain feeling, idea, or suggestion to aid in healing. For cancer pain relief, hypnosis works best when it is added to your medical treatments.

Imagery: A method in which the person focuses on positive images in his or her mind. It may help the body heal or make you feel calmer.

I.V.—intravenous (in-truh-VEE-nus): It means to get medicine or nutrients into the body through a vein.

Legal power of attorney: You appoint a person to make financial decisions for you when you can't make them yourself.

Living will: A type of advance directive. A living will is a legal paper that lets people know what kind of medical care you want if you are close to death.

Massage therapy: Rubbing different body parts to help you relax and gain a sense of well-being.

Notary public: A person with authority from the court to witness legal papers and signatures.

Oncologist (ahn-KAH-luh-jist): A doctor who specializes in cancer study and treatment.

Oncology social worker: A social worker who specializes in helping cancer patients and their families.

Palliative care (PAL-ee-yuh-tiv): Care given to improve the quality of life of patients with a serious or life-threatening disease. The goal of palliative care is to prevent or treat as early as possible:

- The symptoms of the disease
- Side effects caused by treatment
- Psychological, social, and spiritual problems related to the disease or its treatment.

Also called comfort care, supportive care, and symptom management.

Palliative chemotherapy (PAL-ee-yuh-tiv kee-moh-THAIR-uh-pee): Not meant to be curative, this is chemotherapy that may help to relieve the symptoms of advanced stage cancer.

Palliative radiation (PAL-ee-yuh-tiv ray-dee-AY-shun): Not meant to be curative, this is radiation therapy that may help to relieve the symptoms of advanced stage cancer.

Palliative surgery: Surgery used to relieve the symptoms of advanced stage cancer.

Recurrence (ree-KUR-ents): Cancer that has come back after a period of time during which it could not be found. The cancer may come back to the same place as the original (primary) tumor or to another place in the body. Also called recurrent cancer.

Relaxation techniques: Different methods, such as deep breathing and relaxing muscles, that are used to reduce tension and anxiety, and control pain.

Remission: When the signs and symptoms of cancer decrease or go away. There may still be some cancer in the body, but there is less than before.

S.C.—subcutaneous (sub-cu-TA-ne-us): It means to get medicine under the skin. Many can be given this way.

Specialist: A doctor who has studied and trained in a certain area of medicine.

Standard treatment: In medicine, treatment that experts agree is appropriate, accepted, and widely used. Health care providers are obligated to provide patients with standard treatment. Also called standard of care or best practice.

Trust: This type of legal document gives your money and possessions to someone else.

Tumor (TOO-mur): An abnormal mass of tissue.

Will: This type of legal document divides your property among your heirs.

Personal Affairs Worksheet

By filling out this worksheet, you can help family members deal with your personal affairs after you're gone. Be sure to let your loved ones know about this list. It will help them cope with your death and find comfort in knowing your needs and wishes were met. Try to keep it updated and in a safe place. Make sure that only those you trust have access to it.

Banks, savings and loans

Contact Information _____

_____

_____

What Needs to be Done _____

_____

_____

_____

Life insurance company

Contact Information _____

_____

_____

What Needs to be Done _____

_____

_____

Health insurance company

Contact Information _____

_____

_____

What Needs to be Done _____

_____

_____

Disability insurance company

Contact Information _____

_____

_____

What Needs to be Done _____

_____

_____

Homeowners' or renters' insurance company

Contact Information _____

_____

_____

What Needs to be Done _____

_____

_____

Burial insurance company

Contact Information _____

_____

_____

What Needs to be Done _____

_____

_____

Unions and fraternal organizations

Contact Information _____

_____

_____

What Needs to be Done _____

_____

_____

Attorney

Contact Information _____

_____

_____

What Needs to be Done _____

_____

_____

Accountant

Contact Information _____

_____

_____

What Needs to be Done _____

_____

_____

Executor of the estate

Contact Information _____

_____

_____

What Needs to be Done _____

_____

_____

Internal Revenue Service

Contact Information _____

_____

_____

What Needs to be Done _____

_____

_____

Social Security office

Contact Information _____

_____

_____

What Needs to be Done _____

_____

_____

Pension or retirement plans

Contact Information _____

_____

_____

What Needs to be Done _____

_____

_____

Department of Veterans Affairs

Contact Information _____

_____

_____

What Needs to be Done _____

_____

_____

Investment companies

Contact Information _____

_____

_____

What Needs to be Done _____

_____

_____

Mortgage companies

Contact Information _____

_____

_____

What Needs to be Done _____

_____

_____

Credit card companies

Contact Information _____

_____

_____

What Needs to be Done _____

_____

_____

All other lenders

Contact Information _____

_____

_____

What Needs to be Done _____

_____

_____

Employer

Contact Information _____

_____

_____

What Needs to be Done _____

_____

_____

Faith or spiritual leader/organization

Contact Information _____
_____
_____

What Needs to be Done _____
_____
_____

Safety deposit box keys and box location

_____
_____
_____
_____
_____
_____
_____

Safe, lock combinations

_____
_____
_____
_____
_____
_____
_____

Location of other important items (such as jewelry)

_____
_____
_____
_____
_____
_____

Notes

Notes